OVERCOMING
HEADACHES
and
MIGRAINES

LISA MORRONE, P.T.

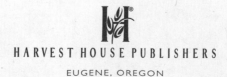

HARVEST HOUSE PUBLISHERS

EUGENE, OREGON

Cover by Koechel Peterson & Associates, Inc., Minneapolis, Minnesota

Cover photo © Agnieszka Pastuszak-Maksim / iStockphoto; interior photos and back-cover author photo © Peter Morrone

Illustrations by Rose C. Miller

Lisa Morrone is published in association with William K. Jensen Literary Agency, 119 Bampton Court, Eugene, Oregon 97404.

OVERCOMING HEADACHES AND MIGRAINES
Copyright © 2008 by Lisa Morrone, P.T.
Published by Harvest House Publishers
Eugene, Oregon 97402
www.harvesthousepublishers.com

Library of Congress Cataloging-in-Publication Data

Morrone, Lisa, 1967-
Overcoming headaches and migraines / Lisa Morrone.
    p. cm.
ISBN-13: 978-0-7369-2169-5 (pbk.)
ISBN-10: 0-7369-2169-9 (pbk.)
1. Headache—Popular works. 2. Migraine—Popular works. I. Title.
RC392.M72 2008
616.8'491—dc22
                                                                    2008002132

Printed in the United States of America

08 09 10 11 12 13 14 15 16 / BP-SK / 11 10 9 8 7 6 5 4 3 2 1

To my husband, Peter—This book has been made complete by your hard work, care, and concern for its every detail. You are a wonderful first-line editor, photographer, encourager, and all-around "Help, I'm having a problem with my computer!" guy. I love you, and I am blessed to be your wife.

_____

To my children, Casey and Adam—Thank you for giving up many a Saturday with Mom and Dad because we were "busy working on Mom's book." I am proud to watch you both take on the character of your heavenly Father as you grow in Him. Thank you for being so patient. Your prayers helped make this book a reality.

_____

To my "headache mentor," Dr. Howard Makofsky—It was back in 1989 when you first taught me about the neck and its involvement in headaches. In so doing, you lit a fire under me that continues to burn today. Thank you for sharing your resources with me as I wrote this book.

_____

To my dear friends—I am forever grateful to you for your faithfulness in upholding me and this book in your prayers.

_____

To those who have shared their personal headache accounts and journeys to healing within this book—Thank you for opening up a window into your lives so others may find hope and healing by identifying with your words.

_____

To Jesus Christ, my Lord and Savior—You have blessed me with the ability to acquire and clearly communicate my knowledge. Thank you for continuing to provide me opportunities to educate patients, colleagues, students of physical therapy, and now the many readers of this book. May the hope and healing I offer them always be sprinkled with your Hope and Healing. To God be the Glory, great things He has done!

CONTENTS

Foreword

by Dr. Howard W. Makofsky

Headache is the third most common cause of missed work, and it affects every area of a person's life," say world-renowned headache experts William Young, MD, and Stephen Silberstein, MD. How sad that millions of individuals around the globe are taking medicine to do nothing more than cope with chronic headaches, when many of these may respond to the types of physical treatments covered in Lisa Morrone's *Overcoming Headaches and Migraines*.

A mentor of mine once said, "Medical conditions should be treated medically and physical problems should be treated physically." As a physical therapist, researcher, and professor, I congratulate Lisa for providing chronic headache sufferers with the physical self-help tools necessary to manage and relieve their chronic pain. This offers hope to people who are many times resigned to a life of silent suffering and despair.

Why exactly is this news so good? There is scientific evidence suggesting that not only neck-based headache (cervicogenic headache), but also tension-type headache—the most common form of chronic primary headache—are correlated to *forward head posture, myofascial trigger points,* and *weakness of the deep neck flexor muscles.* Though you may not be familiar with all these conditions, they are common among headache sufferers—and all of them are treatable! There are some who suggest that even migraines are contributed to by these physical impairments and are therefore treatable using the techniques described in this book.

For these reasons and others, *Overcoming Headaches and Migraines* is a gift, not only to headache sufferers, but also to those in the health professions who are committed to helping them.

—Howard W. Makofsky, PT, DHSc, OCS
Former Co-Director, Headache Center,
Southside Hospital, Bay Shore, New York
Associate Professor, New York Institute of Technology
Adjunct Professor, Touro College
Clinical Assistant Professor, SUNY Stony Brook

Pain, Pain, Go Away...

You can feel it coming on again. Mild as it may be now, history tells you it's going to get worse before it gets better. Just the thought of it tenses your shoulders and sets your jaw. What *won't* you get done today? How bad will the pain get? Will you be able to do anything to change it?

As you ponder these questions, you feel your eyelids lowering to half-mast. Every time a headache occurs, your entire head and face want to "draw the blinds and close for business." Headache is unique that way. Unlike back, neck, shoulder, or knee pain, it has a "power down" affect on its victims. Voice tone changes, eye brightness dims, facial expressions dampen, and attention is directed from the people and tasks before you to the storm swirling through your head. Every simple thought or small movement of your head, neck, or face intensifies your pain.

The statistics on headaches are staggering. As many as 45 million Americans have chronic, severe headaches that can be disabling, according to the National Institute of Neurological Disorders and Stroke (NINDS) and the American Council for Headache Education (ACHE). In a 2004 survey, the U.S. Centers for Disease Control found that the percentages of persons aged 18 to 64 who had suffered from either a severe headache or migraine in the prior three months looked like this:

18-44 years old	18%
45-54 years old	17%
55-64 years old	12%

Headaches result in more than 8 million doctor visits per year in the United States. *One billion dollars* are spent annually on over-the-counter headache medication! And migraine sufferers alone lose more than 157 million workdays annually because of headache pain. As you can imagine, that is a tremendous loss in productivity.

Though you are in the company of many others, you may feel very alone in your struggle against chronic, life-altering head pain. Onlookers, even family and friends, want to know why you are so affected by "just a headache." The mild and occasional headaches they have experienced go away 15 minutes after they pop an Advil. Why can't you just do the same? They don't understand—and in their defense, they *can't* understand. A well-known proverb could be restated thus: "Unless you wore my head during my last headache..." Only you will ever experience what *your* headaches feel like.

Life lived with headaches is an experience of head-splitting pounding, viselike pressure, "sharp shooters"—it's enough to make you sick. For some of you, that is just what it does. First, you see a light show (for free), then nausea comes over you and something comes up—literally. Your only hope is, "This too shall pass." You find a dark, quiet room where you can hunker down and ride out the storm. Maybe you'll be able to sleep it off...

Others of you suffer with frequent "traditional" headaches that differ in intensity from day to day. What began as an innocent once-a-week pain interruption has now become a three-to-four-times-a-week intruder. For some of you, multiple headaches per week eventually became steady, constant, chronic headaches. Now, from waking to bedtime you are never without a headache. You are even beginning to forget what it is like to *not* have pain in your head.

One Person's Headache Journey

Bonnie was a typical example of a patient of mine who displayed this progressive, chronic type of headache. She came to me desperate to get rid of the pain in her head. The headaches she had suffered throughout her childhood began to be peppered with migraines every now and then throughout her college years and early adulthood. Two years before, her headaches had gone from occurring a few times a week to remaining constant from morning through night. Worse yet was the pain in the back of her head. It had now spread into her left eye, and she felt a constant, painful throb that increased every time she closed her eye to blink.

Bonnie was at her wit's end. She had been to an ENT (ear, nose, and throat doctor, or otolaryngologist), who had ruled out a sinus problem. She was examined by an ophthalmologist—eye doctor—who assured her nothing was wrong with her left eye. Next she received half a dozen treatments from a chiropractor, who adjusted the joints of her lower neck, but without any change in her symptoms. Frustrated, she decided to manage her own pain the only way she knew how—with over-the-counter medications. Having used these medicines over the span of many months, she was noticing they were becoming less and less effective. She also worried about the effect that taking so much medication would have on her liver. (Maybe this sounds somewhat like your own headache journey.)

Through specially targeted physical therapy treatment and the application of the principles and education found in this book, Bonnie finally discovered the true *cause* of her headaches. Her recovery soon followed. (I will tell more about her discovery and recovery journey in chapter 3.)

More Problems and Consequences

Trauma-based headaches are also common among people I see. Like them, you may have been in a car accident or suffered some type of impact to your head or neck. Right afterward, you were sore. Then slowly your headache was birthed, and over time you have watched it grow. Now it has grown too big to ignore.

Possibly you are like many of my other headache patients, whose headache pain is so predictable they can almost set their watch by it.

You know for a fact that by 10 a.m., tension will begin to build in your neck. And soon your skull will tighten with pain. It may begin as a gentle squeeze at the back of your head, but you know where it will end up by 2 p.m.—right behind your eyes. And when it reaches its final destination, even shifting your eyes from right to left will cause the pressure to escalate. Time to pop some pills.

Something's got to change. Your headaches are significantly altering your life, and in all the wrong ways. While in the midst of a headache you may find you are irritable, less productive at your tasks, having difficulty concentrating, and withdrawing from people. The withdrawal has to do in part with noise avoidance, but it has even more to do with the fact you are feeling crummy overall. It hurts your head to be animated, to talk and to smile. You'd just rather be left alone.

If your headache interferes with sleep, you may be living life rundown and sleep-deprived. You hope people won't judge your continual yawning as boredom or lack of interest on your part. Worse yet, headaches that come and go have created "anticipation anxiety" in you, because you worry about the timing of your next attack. Where and when will the next ambush by the headache monster come? What part of your day—or how many *days*—will you be robbed of before he lets go of your head?

Chronic headaches can most definitely lead to feelings of depression and helplessness. You may have seen countless doctors and other practitioners with no significant improvements...and therefore resigned yourself to the role of headache victim. *There's nothing more I can do. I'll just have to live this way,* you tell yourself.

Equip Yourself for Lasting Change

It's hard to buy your own statement, though—there's got to be *something* you can do. That's why you are now holding this book.

As a physical therapist practicing in the field of orthopedics, I have been treating headache patients for nearly two decades now, using hands-on techniques, exercises, and patient advice and education. The results have been remarkable. Many headache patients are overmedicated, with less than satisfactory results, all because the actual *cause* of their headaches was missed. You will find my approach unique because *it targets often unrecognized headache sources, as well as neck-based triggers that can result in tension-type and migraine headaches.*

No Professional Has All the Answers

Each health practitioner can only use the tools that are in his or her own toolbox. Some practitioners have more tools than others. Others haven't updated their toolbox in quite a while. Some practitioners use tools that are less widely known and may even draw skepticism from those who have "never heard of 'em." And some are just better at knowing which tool to use and when to use it. This goes for medical doctors, physical therapists, chiropractors—you name it.

The practical approach in this book will equip you with simple self-help methods of treating your headaches. Further, most of the headache books available on the market today tell you which medications and injections you should take to *ease* your suffering. I want to show you how to *stop* your suffering! I view medication as a last-ditch effort, not a first go-to. My experience and expertise in the treatment of headache causes referred from elsewhere in the body and neck-based migraine triggers will empower you to make lasting changes for yourself. If you find you need to go beyond self-treatment options, you will find advice about exactly what you should look for in a treating practitioner.

This book is not just an information resource about headaches. You are holding the guidebook to wellness in your hands—actual help, hope, and healing for chronic headaches and migraines.

Part 1

Why Won't My Head Stop Hurting?

Chapter 1

What Kind of Headache Do I Have Anyway?

The study of the origin and life cycle of headaches has left scientists with more questions than answers. Even with the latest high-tech equipment, researchers still fall short in attempting to explain the start-to-finish process. Doctors still don't know exactly why headaches begin and what causes them to stop once they've begun.

The good news is, we don't need to know exactly how the brain processes your headache in order for you to find some relief. And let's think big, beyond finding relief—and more toward finding a lasting cure! In order for that to occur, what we really need to find out first is what *type* of headache you have. Then we can set off on the road that leads toward your own personal headache-treatment plan. The mission of this chapter is to give you enough information to be making your own headache diagnosis. Basic details of headache types will help lead you in one direction or another. Further into this book you will find detailed descriptions of each headache type and a plan of action that can be taken, both by you and by your health providers.

Becoming a "Headache Student"

Certainly not all headaches are the same, so it is vitally important that your headache condition be properly diagnosed. You need to do your part in becoming a student of your own headaches so you will be able either to diagnose yourself or aid your physician in reaching a correct diagnosis. *Accurate diagnosis is key!* For you to become a good headache student, you must know *what* to be observing when it comes to your head pain.

By the way, I suggest you begin keeping a daily headache diary, like the one provided for you on pages 23–24. The good thing about keeping a headache diary is that you don't have to hide it from your siblings. Seriously, if you are like me, your memory of daily events fades with time. Reliable information gathering is very important, so it shouldn't be entrusted to memory alone.

Sensitive Structures

Though much remains unknown, there are some important things that *are* known about head pain. Interestingly enough, your brain itself is incapable of feeling pain (even though during some headaches you feel as though your brain itself is throbbing!). However, scientists have found there are many other structures within your head and neck that are pain-sensitive. These include certain arteries, veins, and nerves of your brain and neck; your brain's coverings (the meninges); the joints of your upper neck; your first cervical (neck) disc; the skin of your scalp; and the muscles of your head and neck. With all these different pain-sensitive structures, no wonder it's taking so long to figure this whole thing out! And for certain types of headaches, science points to the brain's own chemical reactions as the "match that lights the fire."

How often? The first item to observe and document is the *frequency* of your headaches. How often do they occur? How many do you get in an average month? Headaches that occur less than 1 time per month are considered to be *infrequent*. Between 1 and 15 episodes per month categorizes head pain as *frequent*. If you are experiencing more than 15 headaches per month (or constant headache), your condition is viewed as *chronic*.

When and how long? Along with frequency of headache, you want to note the time at which each of your headaches began and the length of time each one lasted (*duration*). This will give clues about which of the types of headache you may be suffering. (Believe it or not, some headaches characteristically begin in the middle of the night or at the end of a workday.) Other headaches have characteristic durations. Documenting duration also shows your physician how much of your life is spent in pain and, therefore, how serious the situation actually is for you.

How intense? Next to note is the *intensity* of your pain. This is easily recorded by using a numerical pain scale of 1 to 10. Thus, "1" is when you just barely perceive a pain sensation, and "10" is an "emergency room" headache. Where does your headache rank on that scale? Document it in your headache diary. (Just to let you in on a secret, if you report to your doctor or therapist that your headache is a 15 on a scale of 1 to 10, they will immediately view you as a "symptom magnifier" and wonder if there is a psychological factor contributing to your headaches—even though you might just be trying to drive home the fact that your headaches are unbearable. So take my advice, stick to the scale.)

Where? *Location* of pain answers three main questions for your health practitioner:

1. Is the problem unilateral (one-sided) or bilateral (both sides of the head)?

2. What structures may be involved in the creation of the headache? (Different structures have the capability of *referring* pain—making pain travel—to different areas within the head and face.)

3. Is there an initiating area of pain which may be acting as a headache trigger (for example, the neck or jaw).

So keep track of where in your head or neck your pain begins and where it spreads to during the course of each headache.

Specific sensation? Another helpful item in diagnosing a headache is something that is referred to as the *quality* of pain. Specifically, does your headache feel like a tight band around your head? Is it a dull ache? A sharp, shooting pain? More of a throbbing sensation? Different types of headaches are associated with different pain qualities, as you will soon discover.

What else? *Other associated symptoms* present are also important for you to note. See if you recognize any of these:

- stiff or painful neck
- nausea
- vomiting
- visual disturbances (flashing, blinking lights, distorted images, and so on)
- sensitivity to bright lights
- sensitivity to loud noises
- sensitivity to certain strong odors
- nasal stuffiness
- runny nose
- eye tearing
- eyelid swelling
- numbness (loss of sensation)
- tingling (pins and needles)
- loss of part of your visual field
- face drooping
- fatigue, yawning, or both
- agitation

By taking care to pay attention to and document any of the above signs and symptoms related to your headaches, you will begin to unravel the mystery of which headache type you suffer from. The better you are at gathering the needed clues, the closer you will be to finding lasting help. The best aid you can bring to a professional who is helping you is your headache history. Come to your physician's or physical therapist's office armed with at least a month of legible, well-taken notes. Any health-care practitioner will be impressed by a "student" who obviously has done their headache homework.

Daily Headache Diary

Day of the month	Intensity (1-10)	Duration (min-hrs)	Location (specific)	Quality (ache, throb, squeeze, sharp)	Associated symptoms (see list below)
1					
2					
3					
4					
5					
6					
7					
8					
9					
10					
11					
12					
13					
14					
15					
16					

A. stiff or painful neck
B. nausea
C. vomiting
D. visual disturbances*
E. sensitivity to bright lights
F. sensitivity to loud noises

G. nasal stuffiness
H. runny nose
I. sensitivity to strong odors
J. tingling (pins and needles)
K. eye tearing
L. eyelid swelling

M. face drooping
N. numbness (loss of sensation)
O. fatigue, yawning
P. agitation
Q. loss of part of your visual field

* Visual disturbances include flashing, blinking lights, and distorted images.

Daily Headache Diary

Day of the month	Intensity (1-10)	Duration (min-hrs)	Location (specific)	Quality (ache, throb, squeeze, sharp)	Associated symptoms (see list below)
17					
18					
19					
20					
21					
22					
23					
24					
25					
26					
27					
28					
29					
30					
31					

A. stiff or painful neck
B. nausea
C. vomiting
D. visual disturbances*
E. sensitivity to bright lights
F. sensitivity to loud noises

G. nasal stuffiness
H. runny nose
I. sensitivity to strong odors
J. tingling (pins and needles)
K. eye tearing
L. eyelid swelling

M. face drooping
N. numbness (loss of sensation)
O. fatigue, yawning
P. agitation
Q. loss of part of your visual field

* Visual disturbances include flashing, blinking lights, and distorted images.

Primary vs. Secondary Headaches

There are so many different types of headaches people experience: the one that comes along with your flu or sinus infection, the "I've had a stressful day" headache, the "sick" or migrainous headache, the "I just got hit in the head with a hard object" headache, the post–motor vehicle accident headache—and let's not forget the hangover headache. Clearly not all these headaches are from the same source. And likewise, they are not treated the same way. The International Headache Society (IHS) has done the tedious task of defining and categorizing these various headaches into manageable *groups* and *types* (see sidebar). This then aids health practitioners and you, the headache sufferer, enormously by pointing treatment in the right direction.

Headache Specialists

The International Headache Society (IHS) is a worldwide group of scientists and physicians who study and analyze available research in the field of headache. From their findings they have created a *headache classification system* (or groups of headache types) based upon the cause and characteristics (signs and symptoms) of each particular headache. Now, these classifications have changed somewhat over the years depending upon the present and agreed upon scientific knowledge at the time of their meetings. In 2004 the IHS updated and revised their list of headache classifications from their previous list, published in 1988. (Of note was the addition of the *cervicogenic headache*, which we will get to later in this chapter.)

The IHS has assigned all headache types, first of all, into one of two groups: *primary headache* or *secondary headache*. In *primary headache*, the headache *itself* is the problem. (No underlying problem exists.) Under the primary-headache banner are four types:

1. The most common is *tension-type headache* (TTH), which is thought to affect 90 percent of all headache sufferers.
2. The second most common is the *migraine headache* (MI).
3. The third is *cluster headache* (CL).
4. The fourth is simply called *other primary headaches.*

Of course each of these types have subtypes, and on and on. Believe me, there is enough classification and information to *give* you a headache! I will give you a brief, painless summary of these different headache types below and then in greater detail in chapters 3 and 8.

Unlike primary headache, *secondary headache* occurs in response to an underlying condition. As you will come to discover, I hold a special interest in the recently classified secondary headache, named *cervicogenic headache* (CH), a headache originating in the neck structures. It is my professional opinion—and that of many of my physical practitioner colleagues—that many of the patients who have been diagnosed with TTH (tension-type headache) actually have CH. For this reason, my intervention for both of these diagnoses is the same. (We'll discuss them together in chapters 3 through 7.)

Other underlying conditions also known to produce headaches are infections, hormone or blood-sugar levels, or emergency situations such as brain aneurysm. These are important enough to spend an entire chapter on, so in chapter 2 we'll discuss possible causes of non-neck-based secondary headaches and what should be done about each one. Also in that chapter, I will give you important information on what I call an "emergency room headache." If you think you might be having one of those, by all means skip ahead! (You can come back to this spot later.)

For now, let me acquaint you with the three main types of primary headache, as well as my featured secondary headache, the cervicogenic headache. Maybe you will begin to recognize yourself in one of the following personal accounts.

Tension-type Headache

The day started like any other day, up at 6:30 A.M. to shower and get ready for work. I got the kids off for school and sat down to look over my Day-Timer. I already knew this day's schedule was going to be heavy. So I had to plan well to fit it all in. As I pulled out my chair, I noticed my son had left his lunch box on the floor in his hurry to run out the door. Well, add a stop to his school on the way into work. When I had an idea of what my day needed to look like, I packed up my own lunch and headed out (with a stop to drop off the orphaned lunch box).

I arrived at work five minutes late and walked into the waiting room to see that both my 9:00 and 9:30 appointments had shown up at the same time. Juggling, I treated them both, and the day's busyness just escalated from there. One of my patients showed up doubled over in pain (and late—which meant I had more to do in less time). With each appointment I felt my shoulders and neck tensing up more and more. I was falling hopelessly behind that morning, and now some patients were giving me an attitude. Stacked on my desk was a large pile of patient charts and insurance paperwork that would have to wait until the end of my day. By the time I got to write my treatment notes, I could feel a low-level squeeze developing around the circumference of my head. Great, a headache was brewing!

I left work late (what a surprise) and headed directly to the supermarket. Could I shop and be home before my kids' bus arrived back? I raced through the aisles, quickly making my selections, stood in a long line to pay, loaded my groceries into the trunk, and slid into the driver's seat. Exhaling slowly, I noticed my shoulders were not lowering as I breathed out. I was stressed out. And wow, was my head hurting! It felt as if someone had it pressed in a vise.

—M.U.

In a tension-type headache, it was traditionally believed that *tension*, or increased muscle tone, in the head or neck was *the* cause. In fact, when originally classified, TTH was given the name "muscle tension headache," and then later "tension headache." As time went on, new studies failed to find a greater amount of tension in the muscles of the neck and head of a TTH sufferer than in those of their migraine-suffering counterparts. Still, without any other "cause" to point to, the IHS simply added a clarifying (or vague) word to the name: tension-*type* headache. (This was because patients were still reporting "tension" preceding their headache events.) Today the word *tension* has a broader definition. It includes both emotional tension—stress, anger, anxiety—and physical tension—bad posture, faulty ergonomics, neck injury, hunger, and fatigue.

While scientific researchers still have yet to define the exact cause of TTH, enough evidence exists to suggest that some of the brain's chemical changes are similar to those noted in migraine sufferers. This points to a possible brain-based pain syndrome. Even so, it is commonly accepted that neck dysfunction, posture, and positioning can be major triggers for TTH. And by addressing these specific areas, TTH can be made a thing of the past.

Now let's look at the characteristics of TTH to see if they might describe your headache type. The following list describes the common signs and symptoms.

Characteristics of tension-type headache:

- bandlike, bilateral squeezing, pressing, or tightening around the head
- lasts from 30 minutes to 7 days
- mild to moderate intensity (1 to 6 on a "10" scale)
- preceded by tightness in the neck muscles
- neck, scalp, or jaw muscles, or a combination of them, are tender to the touch
- may be relieved by the use of over-the-counter medications
- usually not physically debilitating

Migraine Headache

Migraine headaches seem to have always been a part of my life. My earliest memory of getting an "I'd rather be dead" headache was when I was nine years old. Although I cannot recall the exact nature of my first headache (what it felt like, how it started, and so on), I've had hundreds of migraines over the years and can fill in the details now with certainty. As I went through adolescence, it appeared that my headaches were "cyclical" and related to my menstrual cycle. No one ever called them "migraines" back then (1970s), but in hindsight I am sure that is what they were.

I would get them sporadically throughout my late teens and into my twenties.

By the time I hit my late twenties, migraines were becoming a regular part of my life. Typically, they would start with a subtle tightness on one side of the back of my head. (It took me a while to recognize this symptom as the beginning.) From there, they would progress to a vise-grip, throbbing headache that seemed to pulse behind my eye. Because my migraine headaches had increased in frequency, my doctor gave me some medication (Fioricet) to have on hand. When a migraine would strike, I would take my medication, get an ice pack to put over my eyes, and try to sleep. Most times this did the trick.

However, there have been multiple occasions over the years where the headaches did not respond to medication and I would get to the point of throwing up. Once this happened, it became a very difficult cycle to break. The more I threw up, the worse my headache would become; the worse my headache became, the more I threw up. I was miserable! When I couldn't get out of this cycle, my husband would eventually take me to the emergency room.

I wasn't looking for a diagnosis. I was there for one reason only... for the drugs—anything to stop the pain and nausea! The physicians in the emergency room always gave me a "cocktail" of an anti-nausea drug and a painkiller of some kind (usually Demerol). This usually allowed my body to relax enough (yes, I slept!) for the cycle to be broken. But even though the headache and nausea would stop, the entire episode really took a toll on my body, and it literally took a couple of days to feel like myself again.

—F.M.

People diagnosed with migraine headaches make up a much smaller percentage of the overall headache population than do those with TTH. Even so, there are approximately 33 million Americans who endure them. Migraines are an entirely different animal from TTH. Those who suffer with them even have a chic French name: *migraineurs* (pronounced "mee-gren-ERS").

In 1993 the world of suffering changed significantly for migraineurs. That was the birthday year of the first effective abortive medication available for the treatment of acute migraine. (*Abortive* means "tending to cut short.") Its name? Imitrex. This was a truly exciting day for migraineurs as well as for their doctors—who up to that point had been struggling to help their patients. Finally, some relief!

Another area of excitement in the treatment of migraines is not so new to me or to my fellow manual therapy practitioners. But many migraine-treating neurologists are just starting to discover the effectiveness of manual physical therapy treatment of the upper neck. I have long been amazed at the clinical success I've had when treating migraine patients who have upper-neck problems. For many migraineurs, these problems act as a noxious stimulator for their headaches. Once the issues are corrected, the neck no longer "strikes the match" to ignite their migraines. All this without medication! As you can tell, I'm excited—it may be *you* who can be helped by this intervention. (Look for more information on treatment of upper-neck dysfunction in chapters 4 through 7.)

Migraines are very complicated and diverse. Though they are associated with four distinct, progressive phases from start to finish—phases that are well defined and documented—only 20 percent of migraineurs actually experience all four stages. Below you will find a basic description of what a migraine episode *might* look like (with much more information in chapters 8 through 11). Remember, since you are attempting to determine a *probable* diagnosis for yourself here, see if these headache characteristics describe your own *in general*.

Characteristics of migraine headache:

1. Prodrome
   - sensitivity to light, sounds, or smell
   - stiff neck
   - fatigue
   - anxiousness
   - food cravings

- occurs hours to one full day before aura/headache phases

2. Aura (present in only 20 percent of cases)
- visual disturbances
- light and noise sensitivity
- nausea, vomiting, or both
- lasts less than 60 minutes

3. Headache
- moderate to severe intensity (5 to 10 on a "10" scale)
- unilateral (one side of the head)
- pulsing quality
- pain increases with activity
- lasts for between 4 to 72 hours (that's three days)

4. Postdrome
- fatigue, listlessness, no "get up and go"
- euphoria (It's over, thank God!)

Cluster Headache

I left the job early that day. All I know is, I was feeling "off." I didn't want to fall from the roof of the house I was working on that day. I figured the heat had gotten to me or something. When I got home I went straight to the fridge to get something cold to drink. Then it hit me. A pain in my right eye so sharp I couldn't stay still! I began pacing from one end of the kitchen to the other with my hand over my eye. I was shaking and sweating...and *hurting!*

My wife walked in with groceries in her arms, took one look at me, and dropped her bags on the table. "Honey, what happened to your eye? It's swollen—you look like you were in a fight!" I could barely talk, the pain was so bad. "Just take me to the hospital," I said. During the drive there I wanted to climb out the window. I just shook my legs and kept my head bent forward. I'm ashamed to say that the thought crossed my mind, *Maybe if I jump out of the car, someone will run over me and end this pain!*

At the emergency room I was evaluated and had numerous tests performed, all of which came back negative. Meanwhile my headache was gone. (It left after about an hour.) The emergency room doctor asked if I had a history of alcohol abuse. I told him that I did, but had been "dry" for over eight years. The doctor believed I was having my first attack of a cluster headache. She said these headaches typically affect men, and often those with drinking problems. I didn't like the name of my diagnosis, 'cause "cluster" meant "a bunch." I was referred to a neurologist for follow-up. Before I got to see him, I had three more attacks. I call them attacks because these ain't no common headaches!

The next two weeks were terrible. I had more of the same headaches, and then one day, as abruptly as they began, they stopped. Now I live in fear for the day they return.

—T.S.

Often, with the first occurrence of a cluster-type headache, as with T.S. above, the victim will run (or be driven) to the emergency room. When I was in physical therapy school, I remember these headaches being called "suicide headaches"—they are so excruciating that people have been known to try to take their own lives just to end the misery.

Cluster headaches are so named because they occur in "clusters." A single headache will last only a brief period of time, but it will then recur multiple times in one day or multiple days in a row. This pattern goes on for months at a time and then stops for up to two years… before sometimes beginning all over again. Though cluster headaches will be addressed in greater detail in chapters 8 through 11, in terms of self-diagnosing, you should be able to either rule in or rule out this monster headache after reading through the descriptive list below.

Characteristics of cluster headache:

- severe intensity (10 on a "10" scale)
- unilateral (one-sided), temple or eye area
- sharp stabbing or burning pain

- eye tearing (same side as pain)
- nose congestion or running (same side as pain)
- eyelid swelling or drooping
- anxious pacing during attack
- from 15 to 90 minutes in duration per headache episode

Cervicogenic Headache

The right side of my neck has always given me problems. For as long as I can remember it has been my "weak link." Lately my neck has been sore more often than not. I find myself constantly rubbing it. One day as I was walking on the treadmill, my right shoulder muscles went into spasm. From there the pain moved up into my neck, and I knew it was time to end my workout. By that evening, I had a sharp pain on the right side of my head and another pain between my right ear and my jaw. The next morning, the head pain was still there. My eyelids felt heavy, and by mid-afternoon the right side of my head felt like it had been hit by a brick! Don't you know, that headache lasted for nearly a week. I went to my physical therapist after that episode. I figured my neck must be getting worse.

—L.M.

As of 2004, the cervicogenic headache classification is new to the International Headache Society's list (see sidebar on page 25). And boy, am I thrilled! From my treating experience, I've known that this has been a source of headache since I first began patient care in 1989. What *cervicogenic* means will give you important insight into where this type of headache originates. *Cervico* describes the cervical portion of the spine or neck area in the body (not the cervix of a woman's anatomy). The suffix *genic* comes from the word *genesis,* which means "the beginning." So if you put it all together, *cervicogenic* means, "a headache that has its origin in the structures of the neck." Most of the time, I will simply refer to it as a *neck headache.* (Simple enough for me…and easier to type!)

Characteristics of neck (cervicogenic) headache:
- one-sided (occasionally both sides)
- mild to severe intensity (1 to 10 on "10" scale)
- tender points in the neck muscles and over the upper neck joints
- can be preceded by trauma to the head or neck
- location: forehead, temples, eye area (can include base of skull/back of head)
- can be disabling, depending on severity

I hope that by now you may have been able to place your headaches into one of the four categories above. I say "your headaches" and not "yourself" because I don't believe your headaches should define you. They are something you *suffer with,* they are not *you.* Don't give your headaches any more credit than they deserve!

Some of you may now feel quite certain of which type of headache you have. But others of you may be unsure, even hopelessly confused. No need to be concerned. We've just begun. Several of the upcoming chapters are dedicated to fine-tuning your headache diagnosis. Once your headache type is determined, this book will offer you self-help, hope, and direction toward the management and cure of your headaches.

Chapter 2

Could Something Else Be Wrong?

O ften something else is going on within your body that is causing your headaches to occur. *Secondary headaches* are caused by some underlying medical condition. Some of their causes develop slowly over time, while others present themselves quite abruptly and forcefully. With these latter headaches, immediate action is often warranted.

Case in point: I had been treating Matthew twice a week for three years for a progressive muscular disease. If not for treatment, he would have lost his ability to walk on his own a long time previous. His dry sense of humor and love for classical music were supported by his intelligence. We shared many of the same political and moral viewpoints and often had intense conversations.

When Matthew's 90-year-old mother passed away, it sent him into a "mental funk." His wife called me and said he was in a state of confusion. He visited his doctor and even spoke with a psychologist, who tried to reorient him. The confusion lasted for three weeks time and stopped as abruptly as it had begun. Matthew returned to therapy, weakened for having missed so many treatments.

Two weeks later he arrived with his head hung low. He was not in a joking mood. He pointed to his right temple and said, "Lisa, I've been having the worst headache right here for the past four days." "Did you take any medicine for it, like Tylenol or Motrin?" I queried. "Yes, I did." "Did it make any difference at all?" I probed. "No, not at all," he said. Matthew had never complained of headaches before: he was in his 60s and had recently had that bout of confusion. I turned to his wife, who was in the room, and said, "I'd have that checked out as soon as possible." Sadly, it was discovered that he had a large brain tumor, which despite emergency surgery and chemotherapy, took his life within four months.

I share this story to give you a sense of urgency if you notice any of the following red flags either in yourself or in someone you care about.

WHEN TO SEEK *IMMEDIATE* MEDICAL ATTENTION:

1. You are experiencing "the worst headache you've ever had."
2. The headache has a sudden onset (peak intensity within seconds to minutes).
3. You are over 55 years old.
4. The pain is associated with a stiff neck or high fever.
5. You have no history of headaches, and your first one is occurring later in life.
6. The headache persists longer than three days.
7. It's accompanied by other neurological changes: double vision, slurring of speech, loss of sensation or weakness, wobbly gait (walking).
8. You're experiencing an altered mental state.

The main causes for these emergency headaches are tumors or brain aneurysms (bulging of a blood vessel's walls). However, less than 1 percent of all severe headaches require emergency treatment, so chances are quite high you will not be in this category.

Less Urgent "Something Elses"

Now that the scary stuff is out of the way, let's look at other possible headache causes. Although these do not constitute an emergency, they will require medical intervention to resolve. Along with a description of the possible problem, I will suggest which medical professional is best at handling that particular issue and what to expect in terms of evaluative procedures to rule out or rule in each headache cause. The great news is, all these secondary headache causes are curable!

Eye Strain

Many times the first sign of weakening vision is headaches. If you have not had an eye exam in over a year, make an appointment. As vision weakens, a person squints to see more clearly. Your "squinting muscles" surround your eyes and your forehead. If they are made to contract (squeeze or squint) continuously, they can begin to cry out in pain—headache pain. You should visit either an *optometrist* or an *ophthalmologist* for a complete checkup. Not only will these doctors evaluate the acuity of your vision, but they will also check for underlying eye diseases such as glaucoma and cataracts.

Thyroid-Hormone Levels

The thyroid gland is an endocrine gland located in the front of your neck. Its hormone regulates your overall metabolism (the rate at which you use your energy sources). In addition to calorie burn, thyroid hormones also regulate your blood pressure, heartbeat, and breathing rates. Headaches have been associated with *low* thyroid hormone levels. Other symptoms associated with an *underactive* thyroid gland include chronic fatigue or tiredness, low body temperature, sensitivity to cold, increased hair loss, weight gain (even in the presence of appetite loss), constipation, depression, dry skin, and muscle weakness. Low thyroid-hormone levels in women can also lead to painful premenstrual periods and difficulty conceiving a child. (I have two friends who were unable to conceive for a long time, until it was discovered their thyroid glands were underactive. Once the hormone was regulated, both friends have conceived without any other medical intervention.)

Hypothyroidism—low level of thyroid hormone—is easily regulated by a medication whose brand name is *Synthroid* (generic is *levothyroxine*). Synthroid is actually a *synth*etic form of thy*roid* hormone. When it is added to your body's own natural, but insufficient, source of thyroid hormone, it returns your body's levels to normal range.

Synthroid comes in many different dosages, however, so there is an experimental period needed to determine the correct one for you. The specialist who is best suited to administer the proper blood tests and prescribe the correct dosage is an *endocrinologist*. Many people who have suffered with headaches and low thyroid-hormone levels find that their headaches "magically disappear" when their hormone levels are normalized.

Blood-Sugar Levels

Your brain has a real sweet tooth—it lives on sugar. When sugar levels circulating in the blood drop below normal, your brain just aches for more (sort of like your kids do the day after Halloween!). Reasons for blood-sugar drop could simply be a missed meal or fasting. If this is the cause of your headaches, simply eat something, and make sure you're more regular with meals or snacks. A more serious situation, however, is that of a diabetic patient who is taking too much insulin, which is overcompensating for their food intake. Many in this situation suffer headaches as a result. If you have insulin-regulated diabetes and are experiencing headaches, please schedule a checkup with your *endocrinologist* to ensure you are keeping your blood sugar in normal range.

Blood Pressure

Normal blood pressure is 120 over 80. These numbers, simply speaking, are a measure of how much pressure it takes to overcome the tension in your vessel walls in order for your heart to pump its blood around your body. If your blood pressure gets too high or too low, it affects the pressure in the blood vessels in and around your brain. Headaches can result. If you don't know what your blood pressure is, a good first visit would be to your *primary care physician* (PCP), who is thoroughly capable of monitoring your blood pressure.

If, however, your blood pressure requires medication, a *cardiologist* would be your physician of choice. There are so many different medications on the market, and a cardiologist is an expert in the field of the heart and circulatory system and the medications used to treat associated diseases.

Your Body Needs Maintenance Too

Please don't neglect your annual checkup with your PCP. They are your first defense against illness and disease. Many go to the doctor only when they are sick. Long-term, this doesn't work. Just as cars need tune-ups and oil changes, your body needs a maintenance schedule of its own. Be good to yourself— make an appointment today.

Nasal or Sinus Problems

Now this area can be tricky. Often I have patients who have been sent to me by their physicians to treat their neck pain. During my evaluation I always ask my new patients about associated headaches. Such was the case the day I evaluated Beth. She had suffered with on-again, off-again neck pain for years. Recently her neck symptoms had become more "on" than off. When I asked the usual question, she responded, "Oh, yes, I have headaches every day. But that's something different. I have sinus headaches," she said as she ran her fingers from the bridge of her nose out across her cheekbones. "How do you know they are *sinus* headaches?" I asked. "Well, they're right over my sinuses, and when I take my sinus medicine, they get much better." I didn't argue with her reasoning, though I thought it might be flawed. I continued and finished my exam.

Two days later Beth arrived for her first treatment. During the treatment, I had her lie on her back while I worked on the muscles of her upper neck with a technique called a *cranial base release*. "That's weird!" she exclaimed. "My sinuses are clearing." I chuckled as I explained to her about the neck's ability to refer pain to different parts of the head. In her case, the referral of pain mimicked sinus headaches. Within the next four treatments, Beth's "sinus headaches" were gone for good.

Some sinus area pain truly is caused by *sinusitis,* an inflammation of the tender tissues that line the inside of the sinus passages. Dr. William Spencer, an *otolaryngologist* (or an ear, nose and throat specialist—an ENT) shared an amazing fact with me as I was researching for this book. He told me that our sinuses make a quart of mucus a day! (Kind of gross if you picture all that mucus in one place!) Why would anyone need that much mucus? Mucus is a much-needed friend because it helps to warm and humidify the air you breathe in, and helps to filter out particles in the air which would not be welcomed in your lungs.

This large amount of mucus must drain out of your sinuses through two small openings on either side and then go down the back of your throat. If there is any obstruction, the mucus will back up and pool in the sinus area. Blockage can occur for a number of different reasons, including swollen sinus linings, polyps (abnormal growths), a deviated septum (a curvature in the "wall" which divides the right ride from left side of your nose), or enlarged adenoids (spongy tissue at the back of the nose and throat that helps to fight off infection).

When blocked mucus sits in a stagnant pool, a sinus infection is likely to begin brewing, and this is another secondary cause of headaches. When sinusitis and sinus infections compress the rich blood and nerve supply in the sinus area, a significant sinus-area headache can result.

If you have pain or pressure between your eyes (at the bridge of your nose) or feel a heavy ache across your cheekbones (under your eyes), I suggest a visit to, again, an otolaryngologist (ENT). This specialist will be best able to determine if you have sinus-based headaches or if your headaches or migraines are simply masquerading as sinus headaches.

Drug Rebound

Substances you take regularly that affect your blood vessels or interact with your brain chemicals can cause what are known as *rebound headaches.* Rebound typically begins as a headache problem from a different source, not as a drug problem. As your occasional headaches become more frequent, you turn to some over-the-counter (OTC) medication such as Tylenol or Advil for relief. For some reason you find yourself taking it more and more often and, oddly, it seems to be less and less affective at relieving your pain. Your brain has developed an affection for the presence of those foreign chemicals. When their level in your body drops, the brain does what it did in the first place to *get* those chemicals—it produces a headache. So you rebound to a headache after you stop feeding your brain its desired diet.

Rebound headaches can also result from the medications your doctor has given you for the treatment of migraines, such as Cafergot or Imitrex. Either way, whether OTC- or prescription-medicine-based, rebound headaches are best managed and resolved under the watchful eye of your *primary care physician* or *neurologist*. The cure will involve a weaning-off period or a cold-turkey method. (The first few days are going to be rough ones—you will be going through a withdrawal of sorts.)

An unexpected source of drug-rebound headaches is the common substance *caffeine*. I know you may never have thought of caffeine as a drug, but it is. It is a stimulant. As part of its stimulating effect on your body, caffeine constricts (narrows) your blood vessels. If your brain has become used to "having the squeeze on," when your caffeine level drops, the tiny blood vessels in your head will swell and set off a headache. Your response, whether you are aware of it or not, is to have another cup of coffee (or cup of tea or can of cola). You feed the brain what it needs and it settles down. No more headache.

Caffeine's ability to ease headache pain is the reason it is an added ingredient in so many headache-combating medications, such as the popular OTC medicine Excedrin. For myself, I am fully aware of my addiction to morning caffeine. If I go past 10 a.m. without a cup of black tea, a dull pounding will begin in my head, and it drives me to drink...a cup of tea, so I can again be pain-free.

Anemia

When you hear of someone who is anemic, what comes to mind? A pale, weakened individual who lacks energy and drive for life? Well, that is not so far from the truth, although there is a large range, from mild to severe, that affects exactly how compromised a person will be. Anemia is a condition caused by a decreased number of red blood cell (RBCs); a decrease of *hemoglobin,* an oxygen-carrying protein found in red blood cells; or both.

Hemoglobin has an iron component that acts to deliver oxygen to all the tissues of your body. When there is a reduction in number of RBCs and therefore hemoglobin molecules, the amount of oxygen delivered decreases. A body that doesn't get the oxygen it needs feels tired. When your brain doesn't get the oxygen it needs, it sends out pain signals (headaches) alerting you to the fact that something is not quite right. Simple blood tests that measure your amount of RBCs and level of circulating hemoglobin can be ordered by your *primary care physician*. Anemia is most commonly the result of 1) excessive destruction of RBCs, 2) blood loss, or 3) inadequate production of RBCs, and treatment will depend upon the cause of the condition.

A Major Mechanical Problem: Temporomandibular Disorder

Your temporomandibular joints (jaw joints) are located slightly in front of your ears, between your earlobe and the opening of your ear (see figure 2.1). If you place your fingertip lightly over this area on one side of your head and open and close your mouth, you will feel the movement. Half of each jaw joint is made up of one end of your jawbone and the

other half of the joint is part of your skull. The muscles that control your jaw when you're chewing, talking, or doing other jaw movements, such as yawning, attach to these bones. One of those muscles extends high up into the temple region of your head and another one wraps itself down along the bottom of your jawbone. Jaw move-

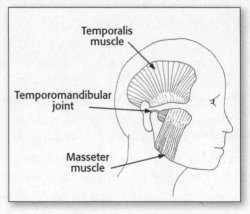

figure 2.1

ments are dependent upon smooth coordination of these muscles as well as how your head sits upon your neck. The temporomandibular joint, being half skull, will be affected if the skull is tipped backward or sits upright on the neck.

My Experience with Treating TMD

Back in the early 1990s I co-directed the Southside Health Institute Temporo-mandibular Joint Center. The other co-director at that time was David Diamond, a doctor of medical dentistry. Together we would evaluate people who were complaining of jaw, head, or neck pain. My task, as a physical therapist, was to examine a patient's jaw and neck muscles and joints for possible dysfunction. Dr. Diamond examined the patient's teeth and bite pattern, looking for possible dental causes for their complaints.

The majority of those diagnosed with temporomandibular joint disorders also complained of headaches. All of these were referred to physical therapy for treatment of their jaw and neck muscles and joints in hopes of relieving their pain complaints. In addition, some patients were referred to Dr. Diamond's office to be custom-fitted with a dental appliance (splint) that adjusted the way their jaw joint was positioned. By the time our patients were discharged from physical therapy, most were headache-free.

During this time I co-authored a specialized home treatment program in *Clinical Management* magazine (March/April 1991). The exercises demonstrated in this article have become an industry standard in the field of physical therapy and are designated by the American Physical Therapy Association as the proper method of home treatment for TMD.*

I've saved this secondary cause of headaches for last because I have a great deal of professional experience with it. (You can read about this in the sidebar.) I believe Temporomandibular joint disorder (TMD) is, today, a commonly overlooked problem in headache diagnosis. Not so 15 to 20 years ago. In the late '80s through the early '90s, nearly every magazine and news program seemed to be asking, "Do You Have TMJ?" Well, it should have been called *TMD,* but though the misnomer stuck around for a decade or so, the information spread about the condition was accurate. TMD sufferers share many of these symptoms: jaw-joint clicking, jaw pain at rest but worsened with chewing, ringing in their ear(s), pain in their face and head muscles, neck pain, limited neck movement, or both.

---

* These TMJ exercises are available for download in a PDF format from my Web site, www.RestoringYour Temple.com.

Health-care professionals enjoyed the increased volume of patients and, unfortunately, some overcharged, overtreated, or actually scammed their patients and their insurance companies out of a lot of money. Finally, the insurance companies put the kibosh on all that treatment spending. As a result, TMJ centers closed, dentists stopped making appliances, and those suffering with TMD had to pay out of pocket much of the expense involved in their care. Along with this came a sense that TMD wasn't a real diagnosis and patients complaining of those symptoms were "symptom magnifiers."

As with most things that are overreacted to, the adjustment was excessive. Somewhere in the middle is the truth. Some patients do have jaw problems, and many of them experience headaches. The first reason is the fact that the jaw joint itself is served by the *trigeminal* nerve, which also supplies the forehead, cheekbone, and jawbone areas (see figure 2.2). Science has demonstrated that pain can carry over from an irritated jaw joint directly into the head and face.

The muscles that control the jaw can themselves create head pain, specifically in the location of the face and temples (above the ear). When muscles are in a state of dysfunction, they often have specific areas of spasm within them. These highly irritable areas are known as *trigger*

points. Not only are these trigger points directly tender to touch, but as their name implies, they can create (trigger) symptoms in another nearby area.

There are two types of trigger points, latent and active. *Latent* trigger points need to be pressed on in order to refer pain to another site. The more severe type is the *active* trigger point. These points are in such a bad

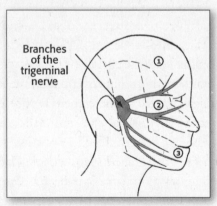

figure 2.2

state that their mere presence refers pain. In figures 2.3 through 2.5 you will find three very telling illustrations, each showing a particular jaw muscle, the location of commonly found trigger points, and the areas to which those trigger points can refer pain. If these muscles are the cause of your secondary headache, only treatment to relieve these trigger points will bring relief to you.

If you suffer with jaw pain, clicking, jaw clenching, or a combination of these, and you also suffer from headaches, there is a pathway to cure for you. First, you should be evaluated and treated by a *physical therapist* who has experience treating TMD patients (this experience is crucial). In addition to the hands-on treatment from your PT, you would greatly benefit from performing the home treatment program I mentioned in the sidebar on page 43.

If you sense your teeth don't fit together right (your bite is "off"), seek help from a *dentist.* Certain dentists still fabricate dental appliances (TMJ splints) for their patients. If you grind your teeth at night, you may need a night guard.* Whatever your course of action, if you feel your headache problems may stem from your jaw, seek help. I've watched many people's headaches fade into nothing with proper treatment of their jaw joints and surrounding muscles.

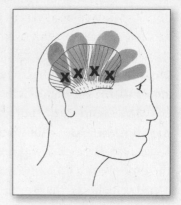

figure 2.3 (temporalis)

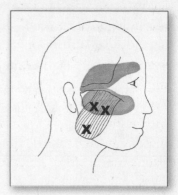

figure 2.4 (masseter)

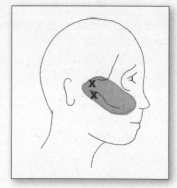

figure 2.5 (lateral pterygoid)

---

* There is an inexpensive, easily customized clenching guard on the market called the NTI. You can find information about it at www.headacheprevention.com.

I hope you are beginning to understand some of the complexity of headache diagnosis after reading these last two chapters. There are so many possibilities among the numerous types of primary and secondary headaches! But hold on to the fact that accurate diagnosis requires 1) a person who has been a good student of his or her headaches, and 2) an informed health-care professional (or two) who takes the time to get a thorough history from you and who performs a complete evaluation to rule in or rule out the many possibilities. And I'm happy to help you navigate through this maze of headache diagnosis.

So far we are off to a strong start. You may already be in the process of making appointments with suggested health-care providers to rule out secondary causes for your headaches. In the upcoming chapters, I want to sharpen your focus on

- three of the most common primary-headache diagnoses, as well as my highlighted secondary headache: neck-based, or cervicogenic
- their causes (as far as is known)
- what you can do about them
- who in the health-care field you should seek help from for them

As we continue examining each feature of these four headaches, I believe your own personal headache diagnosis will likely be unearthed. Then your healing can begin.

Part 2

Headaches That Can Be a Real Pain in the Neck

Chapter 3

Tension-type and Cervicogenic Headaches

The ability for a manual physical therapist to provide a cure for headaches caused by or triggered by the neck is outstanding. Thus I don't see myself in the field of headache *management,* but rather headache *recovery.* Many people have been left to suffer with tension-type headaches and cervicogenic headaches for years, with medication as the only treatment approach offered to them. But more and more research is confirming what manual PTs have known for decades. The physical therapy approach really works!

Now, here's what you'll need to know about neck-based or triggered headaches in order for you to help yourself (and help you spread the good news). While tension-type headaches are highly correlated with neck problems (posture, positioning, dysfunction), cervicogenic headaches are without a doubt *head*aches—but ones that begin in the *neck* before traveling up into your head. They are a prime example of referred pain. A commonly recognized example of this is the left-arm pain that can accompany a heart attack. There is nothing wrong with the heart attack victim's left arm—it's just the way in which the human body is wired.

So it is when it comes to neck-based or neck-triggered head pain. Structures within your neck, shoulders, head, and face areas are wired in such a way that they are often responsible for sending (referring) pain into neighboring areas of the head. When a problem is sensed in one of these "off-site" areas, signals travel up to your head and into your brain along a complex system of nerves built especially for sensing pain. The end result can be 1) blood-vessel swelling in the head or face or across the covering of the brain; 2) nerve inflammation in the head and facial areas; 3) increased tone or spasm in the muscles of your head, neck, and shoulders. All three of these can contribute to your head pain. Because of the great complexity of this wiring, science is somewhat at a loss when it comes to understanding and explaining the exact process of neck-related headache production.

Spreading the Word

The motivation to write this book comes out of my experience with those head-aches that are a real "pain in the neck." As a manual physical therapist I use skilled, hands-on evaluation techniques and treatment approaches with all of my patients. The simple fact is, these techniques and approaches are vastly unknown (until now) to physicians.

Unfortunately, communication regarding treatment advances is poor between the different fields of medicine. This book is offered as a communication-barrier breaker. I want to get the word out, and what better way than to begin with you. (And I can help you at the same time!) Take this information to your next visit with your doctor. Many doctors will be thankful to learn they can offer an alternative plan to their patients who suffer with chronic head pain. And you will have done your good deed for the day.

Find the Source, Define the Treatment

The problem with referred pain is that it often leads to the wrong conclusion. If your left arm aches, you immediately think, *There's something wrong with my arm.* When your head begins to hurt, you very rationally decide, *Something is wrong with my head.* This is why a proper history, evaluation, and examination of a patient, as well as good information, are crucial. For an accurate diagnosis to be made, it is important to first know all the possible causes of pain referral into the area of the body in question. Next, it is important to know how to rule out (or rule in) each possibility. With TTH and CH there are many possible neck-related pain sources or triggers ranging from discs and muscles, to joints and nerves.

By the end of this chapter, you will be able to have a clear understanding of each of the possible neck-pain sources that, given the right situation, can refer pain into your head. *Only when the true pain source is identified can proper treatment begin.* You will also be able to distinguish the unique differences between tension-type headache and cervicogenic headache so you can "name" your neck-related headache. (A comparison chart is located near the end of the chapter.) With an accurate diagnosis in place, you'll be able to help yourself further. Chapters 4 through 6 will show you what you can do for yourself, and chapter 7 will tell you what can be done for you in the hands of a trained physical practitioner. (You will even be equipped, if the need arises, to educate the professionals you seek treatment from about the possible culprits in your headache.)

My understanding of possible head-pain sources comes from widely accepted scientific experiments and studies, as well as my own clinical observations and experiences. *The treatment methods I have used and refined over the last two decades have eliminated the headaches in nearly every neck-based headache patient I have treated!* Before we go through these treatment techniques in the following chapters, let's first make sure you have a full understanding of what you are dealing with in regard to your neck-related or neck-triggered headache.

Tension-type Headaches

My neck pain and headaches began in 1997 after I was involved in a motor-vehicle accident. Immediately following the accident, I thought I was fine. After filling out the police report I went home, shaken but thankful that everyone involved was okay. The next day when I woke, my neck was locked in an extremely painful chin-to-chest position. At that point I was desperate for relief. I called a local chiropractor and made an appointment. The chiropractor, upon examining me, said he really couldn't treat me because my neck muscles were locked in spasm. From his office I went directly to my family doctor, who prescribed muscle relaxers and told me to rest. Unfortunately, the medicine he prescribed severely irritated my stomach, and I was unable to tolerate any other similar medications.

A few weeks later, after I had regained some movement of my neck, I returned to the chiropractor. He applied moist heat packs to my back and neck and made a few adjustments to my spine. It was very relaxing and did help my situation a little. However, after many months I felt frustrated that the time and effort put into the sessions was not producing complete relief from my neck pain and headaches. So I stopped going to the chiropractor.

My life was very busy, filled with the normal craziness of a family, school activities, sport events, meals, entertaining, and medical issues. I thought that if I learned to relax and exercise properly, the headaches and neck pain would go away. However, my neck pain made it difficult to exercise, and the constant nagging headache left me tired and unmotivated. Nothing was improving, and I was increasingly exhausted.

After some time had passed, I returned to my family physician. He prescribed prednisone (an anti-inflammatory) and sent me for an MRI of my neck. The prednisone gave me total relief from my neck pain and headaches for about two months. When the pain returned, I went back to him. It was then that I got the results of my neck MRI. It showed I had a squashed disk, a little arthritis, and a bone spur resting on a nerve. My doctor said that given the findings, there wasn't much that could be done. He said this in a defeated "I'm sorry, you'll have to live with this" manner.

From that point I tried to work through the pain myself. I tried moist heat, I rested, and I even tried to ignore the pain. Each day I would make it until about two in the afternoon, and then I'd have to lie down. My head felt as if it were just too heavy for my neck, and the nagging headache made me so tired. My pain soon became so exhausting and limiting that I returned to my doctor for another round of prednisone and asked for a referral to a neurologist. The neurologist I visited had the same "I'm sorry, you'll have to live with this" attitude. He reluctantly gave me a prescription for physical therapy when I asked for it. But he didn't seem confident it would help any. Boy, was he wrong! (To be continued in chapter 7.)

—W.J.

Ninety percent of all primary headache sufferers are diagnosed as having tension-type headache. (I sincerely believe this percentage includes a large number of misdiagnosed cervicogenic headache patients.) According to the World Health Organization and the U.S. Census clock, 120 million women and 96 million men in the United States suffer with tension-type headache (TTH). That is a huge number of people! Wouldn't it be wonderful if the medical community knew what to do about all those headaches?

What Are TTH's Characteristics?

While treatment options are often unclear, the signs and symptoms of TTH have been well defined by the International Headache Society.

- A typical tension-type headache has been noted to last from *between half an hour to a full week.*
- Pain is experienced on *both sides of the head* simultaneously.
- The quality of the pain is often described as *bandlike—a squeezing or tightening sensation* that encircles the head.
- Most often, patients report *tightness (tension) in their neck muscles* prior to headache onset. When these headache sufferers press their fingertips into the muscles of their shoulders, neck, scalp, or jaw they find specific areas of tenderness.
- Furthermore, tension-type headaches do not have a pulsing or throbbing nature; rather, they feel like a *steady ache.*
- The intensity of these headaches is *mild to moderate,* although they may become severe and even disabling if chronic.
- They are *not typically worsened with activity,* such as walking or stair-climbing. During a single such headache, most people are able to carry on with their daily activities, even though they may be considerably distracted by their pain.

- Unlike migraines, TTH is *not associated with nausea or vomiting*. While there may exist a sensitivity to light or sound, both do not exist at the same time during the same headache.

Quality of life for a TTH sufferer depends much upon the frequency of the headaches. Nearly everyone suffers from an occasional (or infrequent) tension-type headache. By definition

- *Infrequent TTH* amounts to less than one headache per month (which is less than 12 headaches per year). When they occur, you simply pop an aspirin or the like and you are done with it.

- *Frequent TTH* begins to chip away at life. Headaches occur between 1 to 15 days per month for at least three months. Now you find yourself eating through a bottle of Tylenol more quickly, not to mention that your productivity levels begin to slow and your frustration levels are on the rise.

- Life is truly altered when the frequency of your headaches increases to more than 15 headaches per month for a period of greater than three months. When frequency reaches this level, people are diagnosed as having *chronic TTH*. This is the group that most often seeks medical help, usually beginning with a visit to their primary-care physician.

Figuring Out Causes

When chronic TTH patients ask their doctor why they are getting their headaches, they often are told, "You're probably under a lot of stress," or "It may be an accumulation of many factors, such as your prior whiplash injury or the arthritis in your neck." Most likely your doctor is aware that the International Headache Society and every headache book on the market states the "fact" that the cause of tension-type headache is "unknown." So why does he or she offer you these possible reasons? Many doctors don't want to disappoint you. They know you want answers, so they kindly provide you with some. Also, I think that deep down, your doctor (like me) doesn't agree with the "unknown cause" statements regarding TTH.

That said, whenever there is scientific confusion as to the exact cause of a particular type of headache, there also exists confusion as to how to treat it. Traditionally, doctors "treat" their TTH patients with pain medications. This is a cover-up if you ask me. Medication merely relieves pain; it does nothing toward fixing the problem. Head pain remains masked because doctors and their patients are treating head-ache *symptoms* and not the underlying headache *cause.*

Clinically speaking, I have treated countless people over the last 20 years who have come in with classic TTH and who leave, after my course of treatment, *without any headaches.* My manual physical therapy treatment approach does not include psychological counseling or stress management. It simply addresses the problems I discover in my patient's head and neck regions.

Judy, a former TTH patient of mine, is one of many examples. A busy mother and office manager, Judy had begun to get headaches a year earlier. These headaches didn't get her full attention until they became a near daily occurrence. Up to then she had managed to get through her long days by taking extra-strength Motrin. When she got to the point of having to pop a pill every four hours to keep her headaches in check, she finally decided to take care of herself and seek professional help.

Her primary-care physician recommended physical therapy. On the day I evaluated her, Judy's neck muscles were on overdrive. They were tense, tight, and filled with tenderness, as if Judy's head were being held up by a rigid pole. *No wonder she has headaches,* I thought. Over the next month I did my thing (see chapter 7), and Judy followed up with a home program (chapters 4, 5, and 6). Each week she reported decreased headache frequency and intensity. By the time four weeks were over, Judy's headaches were a thing of the past.

This scenario has been repeated in my office so many times that I have become a believer! I can't state it strongly enough: "Head-ache treatment should be offensive and not defensive." Let's not wait around for a headache to occur (or return) and then do something about it (like sweep it under a carpet of ibuprofen). Let's figure out what's causing your particular headache and treat its cause.

It can be done. You can have your life back.

Muscles Gone Bad

Tension-type headaches are often related to problems of the neck that can result in muscle *dysfunction*. Muscular tension in the neck can easily refer pain into the head. This increased tension in your neck muscles can be due to (but is not limited to) trauma; underlying joint or disc degeneration; bad posture; harmful or prolonged positioning of the head, neck, and shoulders; weakness of the deep muscles of the neck and shoulder blades; repetitive injury from bad lifting techniques, the presence of emotional stress; or all of the above. Whew! That's a mouthful. Whatever the cause, science has shown that the resulting muscle dysfunction will include a combination of muscle shortening (tightness) and an increase in overall muscle tone (*tension*, hence the name).

Within a dysfunctional muscle, you can often identify the presence of *trigger points*. As you recall from chapter 2, trigger points are small, focused areas within a muscle that are highly irritated. Tender to the touch, these points have been shown to refer pain to another location in the "surrounding neighborhood" both when simply present and when compressed. *Active trigger points* are "on" all the time. If you are sitting around doing nothing, or if you make a movement that uses the affected muscle, pain will be referred into your head. A *latent trigger point* refers pain only when someone presses on it.

Five key muscles of the neck, when plagued by trigger points, have the capacity to refer pain into the head and face. They are the *upper trapezius* (figures 3.1a and b); the *suboccipitals* (figure 3.2); the *sternocleidomastoid,* or *SCM* for short (figures 3.3a and b); the *splenius capitis* (figures 3.4a and b); and the *splenius cervicis* (figures 3.5a and b). All of these muscles are paired—meaning you have two of them, one on the left side and one on the right. (The suboccipitals are actually a paired group of mini-muscles.) Treatment of these trigger points and the muscles in which they are found is critical when seeking to wipe out tension-type headaches. Each of the muscle illustrations below demonstrates the muscle itself along with the distribution of referred pain (grayed area) from each trigger point (noted by an "X").

Upper trapezius

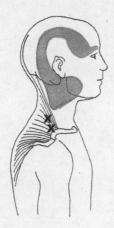

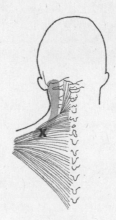

figure 3.1a

figure 3.1b

Suboccipitals

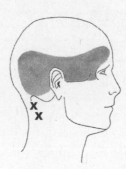

figure 3.2

Sternocleidomastoid

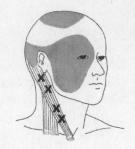

figure 3.3a

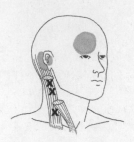

figure 3.3b

Splenius capitis

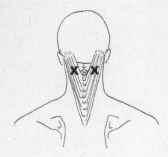

figure 3.4a

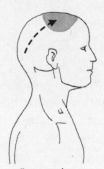

figure 3.4b

Splenius cervicis

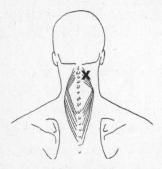

figure 3.5a

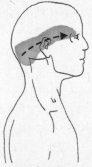

figure 3.5b

Mapping Trigger Points

The scientific research that connected the neck muscles' trigger points with particular areas of pain referral into the head and face was conducted by Janet G. Travell, MD. She first made careful notation of the location of a muscle's trigger points and the area of the patient's associated pain complaint. Next Dr. Travell injected a painkiller directly into the trigger point itself and noted which of the symptom areas were eliminated immediately following her injection. Through this painstaking method she was able to map out diagrams like those above, linking trigger points with specific pain referral locations.

The "why" as to the creation of these trigger points is not completely understood. It certainly varies from person to person. For one it may begin with a muscle strain injury (whiplash), for another an underlying bulging disc—yet for a third it is faulty posture, and for a fourth it is arthritis of the neck. For some it is acute or prolonged emotional stress.

This is when a health practitioner with a full set of tools comes in handy! In the home repair world, a hammer is good to own if you need to bang in a nail. Likewise a Phillips-head screwdriver is a must when trying to sink a Phillips head screw. Sometimes you need to reach for a wrench if you're tackling a stuck bolt. If your health-care practitioner owns only a "hammer," you are at a significant disadvantage. When I seek to eliminate my patient's tension-type headaches through hands-on treatment, exercise, and education, I rely not only upon trigger-point research, but upon the many other tools of physical evaluation and treatment I have "collected" along the way. Only then can I be a well-equipped physical therapist.

There's more good news ahead. In the following chapter you will find a treasure chest of self-help materials, which will address nearly all of the causes of increased muscle tension in your neck. Chapter 7 will then give you a complete "tool list" to look for when choosing a physical practitioner. And I haven't forgotten about the emotional stress you may be experiencing as well. Negative emotions like these certainly have the effect of causing increased tone in the muscles of your head and neck.

Chapter 12—"Navigating through the Seas of Discontent"—will offer helpful advice for dealing with anger and anxiety. If you know these are emotional issues you struggle with prior to getting a headache, by all means jump ahead. I'll meet you back here later.

Cervicogenic Headaches

I am a 31-year-old woman who has been suffering from headaches since childhood. When I was in elementary school I can remember getting a headache two or three times per week. My only defense was spending many hours lying down in a quiet, dark room waiting for the Advil my mom gave me to kick in. The location and quality of my headaches varied from throbbing, pulse-like aching across the left side of my forehead, to sharp, painful twinges in my right temple. My childhood and high school years were filled with many doctor consultations, scans, and tests, which all resulted in inconclusive information as to the reason for my head pain.

After graduating college I began my teaching career. The number of headaches I was experiencing was greatly reduced. I thought maybe I had grown out of my problem. I was wrong. For the past three years my headaches have increased in frequency and seem to be different from the headaches I experienced as a child. My headaches now originate in the back of the left side of my head and upper neck area. In addition to this new "starting position," I have also been experiencing a heavy pain in my left cheek and eye. These pains rise to an acute sharpness and last two to four days before lessening. Although the sharpness of the headache does ease, the dull ache no longer goes away completely. Every day, the simple act of blinking is enough to feel a toothache type of pain in my left eye. The worst thing is that my tried-and-true treatment of taking two Advil and lying down is no longer effective for me.

Concerned by these new symptoms I went to see a dentist, an eye doctor, a chiropractor, and an ENT just to make sure these areas of my body were in good working order. All checked me out and gave me a clean bill of "health." Relieved, yet a bit disappointed, I was once again left without any answers. I didn't know what to do next. So I suffered like this for a year and a half. One day a friend suggested I try physical therapy. I was unsure of what a physical therapist would be able to do, but at this point, I was willing to try anything! (To be continued in Chapter 7.)

—R.W.

As I noted in chapter 1 cervicogenic (neck) headache is the "new kid on the block," in view of its 2004 acceptance as a category by the International Headache Society. Because of this, estimates on the number of people suffering from them have not been published in the literature. Controversy still exists on exactly what defines a cervicogenic headache. Manual physical therapists want to define it by what they feel taking place in the joints and muscles of their patient's necks. Other headache specialists and neurologists want to define it by how the patient's neck moves, what causes the headache to occur, and if the patient's neck muscles are tender to the touch. Pain specialists define a headache as cervicogenic only when they can inject a pain-relieving medication into a joint or nerve in the patient's upper neck area that immediately eliminates their headache complaints.

Characteristics of CH

While the health-care field may still have some diagnostic disagreement, the members of the International Headache Society have agreed upon the common findings (*diagnostic criteria,* as they call it) that, if present, allow a headache patient to be diagnosed as cervicogenic:

- First of all, it was established that cervicogenic headaches show *unilateral pain*—the headache is felt on only one side of the head and does not switch back and forth from right to left with different episodes. (However, they then followed that up with the phrase "occasionally occurring on both sides"! Oh, well.)

- Next it was determined that these headaches were brought on by either *neck movements, sustained awkward head postures, physical pressure held against the back of the head or upper neck, or a combination of these.*

- Signs and symptoms that also must be present in order for this diagnosis to apply are *limited neck range of motion* (movement) and *neck, shoulder, or arm pain on the same side of the headache.*

- "Neck" headaches are *mild to severe* in their pain intensity. The actual pain level (on a scale of 1 to 10) can vary during a headache episode or from one episode to the next. Head-pain quality tends to be a *steady ache* rather than a sharp or throbbing sensation.

- When these patients are examined, they are consistently found to have *tender points in their neck muscles and overlying their upper neck joints.*

All those who study and treat cervicogenic headaches have unanimously agreed upon one thing: the location of the structures responsible for causing cervicogenic head pain. *The origin of the cervicogenic headache is within the upper cervical spine, specifically from the level of the C3 vertebra up to the base of the skull* (figure 3.6). This small area of the neck contains *five joints,* the *C2-C3 disc,* a number of important *muscles* responsible for head on neck control, and *three paired spinal nerves:* C1, C2, and C3 (all of which exit the spinal cord at their named levels and travel directly upward into the back of the head). These structures are intimately connected with your spinal cord,

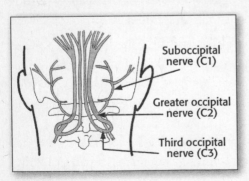

your brain, and the nerves supplying sensation to your head and face. Scientific studies have proven that each one of these structures, when aggravated, has the potential to refer pain into your head or face or both.

The process of how your upper-neck dysfunction can

figure 3.6

become a headache is complex. Allow me to simplify it for you (and for me) with the analogy of a railroad map. Look over figure 3.7 first (see next page), and then we'll talk about it. Here a picture truly is worth a thousand words!

The Neck-to-Head-Pain "Train Map"

Each of the possible head-pain sources in the neck send their pain messengers into the head by way of "pain tracks" (we'll call them "train tracks"). When one of the six spinal nerves in the upper neck (C1, C2, and C3, each paired on the right and left sides) picks up a signal that something is wrong, pain messengers begin to board the "Pain Train," located in the spinal cord. Their only objective at this point is to travel north—toward the head.

The first stop on the Northern Line is the "TCN (don't ask!) Junction Station," which is also located within the spinal cord of the upper neck. At this junction, your pain messengers have a choice to make. They can continue riding north on the "Neck Line," or they can transfer to the "Head Line," which likewise

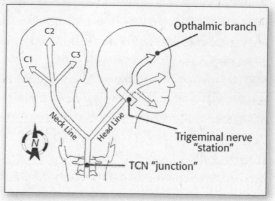

figure 3.7

leads north. The Neck Line, if taken, immediately divides into three branches: the C1 (suboccipital nerve), the C2 (greater occipital nerve), and the C3 (third occipital nerve). The three "stations" serviced by the right and left C1, C2 and C3 branches are located across the back of your head (the *occiput*).

Pain messengers that transfer to the Head Line will find that, though it has a number of smaller branches, its main branch is the *trigeminal nerve*. The "Trigeminal Branch" soon divides into three branches of its own, any of which your pain messengers can choose to continue traveling on. That said, most of them opt for the "Ophthalmic (or eye area) Branch." The Ophthalmic Branch then transports pain messengers to a final "station" and lets its passengers off in the neighborhood surrounding the eye, forehead, and temple.

The location of your neck-based head pain is determined by the final destination of the train ride. If your upper neck's pain messengers choose to ride north along one of the branches of the Neck Line, their final "stop" will be at the back of the head (which is supplied directly by the C1, C2, and C3 spinal nerves). If, on the other hand, your neck's pain messengers decide to transfer at the TCN Junction Station and take a ride on one of the Head Line's branches, then you will feel pain in one of the regional "stations" associated with that particular branch. For example, if the Ophthalmic Branch is chosen, you very well might be feeling pressure behind your eye or across your forehead. Now, remember from figure 3.6 that each of these spinal nerves is paired (one on the right, one on the left). As a result, cervicogenic head pain will be specific to the side of your body from which the pain message was originally sent. Therefore, a right-sided neck signal will produce pain in the right side of your head. Certainly you can have pain messages which originate from both sides of your neck and in that case, have head pain on both sides as well.

The Pain Train Map above and my explanation may need some extra time to digest. If the process of pain referral from the neck into the head interests you, take some time to reread it and understand it more thoroughly. If it doesn't seem of particular importance to you, let's move on.

What "Lights the Fuse"?

Now, let's return to the neck, by definition the origin of neck-based headaches. It's time to switch to a somewhat different analogy to explain the *specific problems* that may be causing your cervicogenic headaches. (Remember, unless the specific cause is detected, no cure will be found.)

Think of your head pain as a stick of dynamite. We'll consider the paired C1, C2, and C3 spinal nerves to be three possible "fuses" that can lead to your cervicogenic headache "blast." There are a number of possible "matches" in your upper neck that, when "struck," can set fire to one of your spinal nerve fuses. The chart below reveals the "book of matches" in your upper neck. It takes only one match to light one fuse on one side of your neck to lead to a one-sided cervicogenic headache. (To avoid too much detail, the chart includes only the structures you've seen in figures 3.1 through 3.6.)

"Matches"	C1 Spinal-nerve Pair "Fuse"	C2 Spinal-nerve Pair "Fuse"	C3 Spinal-nerve Pair "Fuse"
Muscle (dysfunction)	Suboccipitals (right or left)	Sternocleidomastoid, Upper trapezius (right or left) Splenius capitis and cervicis (right or left)	Splenius capitis and cervicis (right or left)
Joint (restricted movement or arthritis)	C1-C2 C0-C1 (right or left)	C1-C2	C2-C3 (right or left)
Spinal disc (degeneration)			Bulging or herniation of the right or left side of the C2-C3 disc

After I explain my match-and-fuse analogy to my cervicogenic headache patients, I get right to work on their upper necks. Again and again, as I press my fingers into a muscle spasm or try to move a stuck joint, they respond with "That's making my headache better!" or "That's making my headache worse!" To both remarks I say, "Good! At least now we know where your headache is coming from." Belief (in my analogy) and relief (because they have finally found someone who knows how to fix their headaches) sweep over them. I can see it in their faces.

Allow me to recap, since this chapter has contained much information that is probably new to you. Tension-type headaches and cervicogenic headaches are often (in the case of TTH) or always (in the case of CH) born out of *neck* problems. TTH can be triggered by excessive tension in the muscles of *the neck as a whole,* stemming from either emotional or physical stress. CH's root problem more typically lies within the joints, disc, or muscles of the *upper neck* (or a combination of them). While both TTH and CH can stem from similar neck-related problems, they do have some distinctive symptomatic features that set them apart from one another, as the comparison chart below shows.

Tension-type Headache	Cervicogenic (Neck) Headache
Both sides of head	One side of head
Increased tone in all muscles of the neck	Pain present in same-side neck, shoulder, or arm
Mild to moderate intensity	Mild to severe intensity
"Band-like" squeezing, encompassing pressure	Localized, steady ache in one or more areas of the same side of the head
Not worsened with activity	Worsened with neck movements, awkward head postures
Neck, scalp, or jaw muscles tender to the touch	Same-side area(s) of upper neck tenderness

The pain-triggering areas in the head, neck, and shoulder regions can result from trauma, such as whiplash, or from bad posture, an overuse injury, or even emotional stress. No matter the initial cause, treatment is needed.

After reading this chapter you may be almost certain your headaches are neck-based or neck-triggered. What should you do about it? Well, if you read the next chapter, you'll learn how you can help (and hopefully fully resolve) your neck-related headaches. If you can't do it all on your own, chapter 7 will describe the practitioner whose skills will do the trick. So let's move on!

Chapter 4

Do-It-Yourself: Healing Through Posture Changes

Welcome to the first of three do-it-yourself chapters for neck-related headaches. Why "do-it-yourself"? Because from my experience, I trust in your ability to heal your own headaches. You just need some direction. Time and time again I have witnessed rapid improvement in people's headaches when they apply different combinations of these DIY exercises and lifestyle modifications.

How should you approach this material? Well, the only way to know which combination will unlock your headaches is for you to try them all, one section at a time. But take it easy—don't apply everything in the DIY chapters at once. Make modifications to your posture and activity positions first, and then progress through each following section. You needn't stop performing the activities of an earlier section in order to apply the guidance of later ones. Allow them to build on one another. By making these key improvements, your headaches will become less intense and less frequent with each passing day. In the end I hope your headaches will be nothing more than a bad memory!

Healing Postures

For many of you, the way in which you stand, sit, and sleep puts you at risk for developing headaches. If you don't pay attention to how your head is positioned in relation to the rest of your body, you in effect "do yourself in." Headaches that are set off by improper posture can often be eliminated simply by making the changes below. It can be that easy!

A New Picture for Standing and Sitting

I like to picture the body as a series of "blocks" that are stacked, one upon the other, to form a "block tower." Your feet are the first block, your hips the second, your shoulders the third, and your head is the fourth and final block in the stack. The way in which you position (or stack) your first through third blocks has a significant impact on the position of your head block, thus affecting its resting position.

Basically, your head is the last "block"—it rests at the top of your body's "block tower." The stacking position of the blocks below— the blocks of your spine—has a definite effect on how your head is positioned at the top. If your low back is flat (no arch) and your shoulders are slumped forward, then your "head block" will tip backward on your "neck block" (see figures 4.1 and 4.2b). Your head does this backward tipping so your eyes can continue to look straight ahead. (If your head followed the forward-bent curve of your slumped shoulders, you'd spend your day looking at the ground in front of you.) If, on the other hand, your shoulders are drawn back, your head block will sit in an upright, slightly chin-tucked position on your neck (see figures 4.1 and 4.2a).

Standing

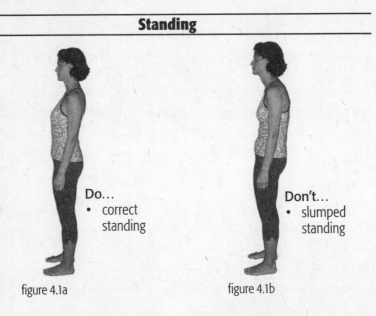

Do...
• correct standing

Don't...
• slumped standing

figure 4.1a   figure 4.1b

Why is this upright position desirable for you as a headache sufferer? Remember all the possible neck-based headache "fuses" (chapter 3) located in your upper neck? If your head has to tip backward in order to keep your eyes level or looking straight ahead, excessive backward-bent stresses are placed on your upper neck. Subsequently, your spinal nerves become compressed, your upper-neck muscles shorten, and your joints experience abnormal compression forces. Prolonged backward-bent head positioning can also result in disc degeneration within the neck. Who knew holding your head in a poor position could be so harmful? I've had many patients who, just by sitting up straight, have immediately lessened their headache intensity by a third or more. Go ahead, give it a try!

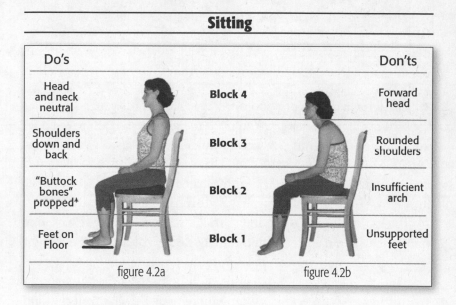

Sitting

Do's		Don'ts
Head and neck neutral	Block 4	Forward head
Shoulders down and back	Block 3	Rounded shoulders
"Buttock bones" propped*	Block 2	Insufficient arch
Feet on Floor	Block 1	Unsupported feet
figure 4.2a		figure 4.2b

New Pictures for Sleeping

Do you wake up in the morning with a headache? The way you are sleeping could be to blame. Good sleeping posture is all about the

---

* In order to maintain an effortless low back arch, try sitting on a wedge-shaped cushion like the one shown above. These cushions are available at my Web site, www.RestoringYourTemple.com.

pillows: how many you use and where you put them. Sleeping on your back needs only a few minor adjustments to make it a healthy head and neck posture. Simply place one pillow under your neck and head (figure 4.3a), *not* under your shoulders and head (figure 4.3b). This pillow placement prevents your head from backward bending on your neck all night. Therefore you avoid compressive injury to the nerves, muscles, disc, and joints in your upper neck.

Do...
• support your head and neck

Don't...
• support your shoulders
• result: your head will tip backward

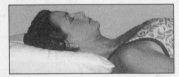

figure 4.3a

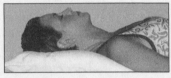

figure 4.3b

Side-lying is a great position for sleeping as long as you, again, have the proper pillow placement. You need to have enough pillow support under your head in order to keep your nose in line with your breast bone (See figures 4.4a, b, and c). This way the joints, muscles, and discs in your neck remain in healthy, centered alignment throughout the night. No more waking up with a stiff neck and headache!

The last sleep position to mention is stomach-sleeping. I have one thing to say if you are a convinced belly-sleeper: please stop! All night long you're stretching, compressing, and twisting your neck to the max and then leaving it like that for eight hours. Oh, the damage you are causing to your neck! How can you remedy this harmful position and still get a good night's sleep?

Presenting...the modified stomach-sleeping position. That's right, *modified*. Begin by setting yourself up as though you were going to sleep in a side-lying position. (A body pillow works best here.*) Use one

---

* Body pillows can be purchased through my Web site, www.RestoringYourTemple.com.

pillow under your head, which should support your head only from your ear to the back of your head. In other words, allow your face to hang off the edge of the pillow (figure 4.5).

Next, turn the front of your body toward the mattress, straightening your bottom leg and sliding it out from beneath the body pillow. Your top leg and your trunk will be supported by the body pillow, and your head will be turned about 45 degrees toward the mattress, as opposed to 90 degrees when stomach-sleeping. This modified position gives you the *feeling* of full-front contact with your sleeping surface. Now you can sleep comfortably without stressing out your neck.

Daily Deeds That Lead to Your Undoing

Throughout your day you carry out some tasks that require you to remain stationary and other tasks that send you moving about. You are either still or you are moving (how's that for an obvious statement?).

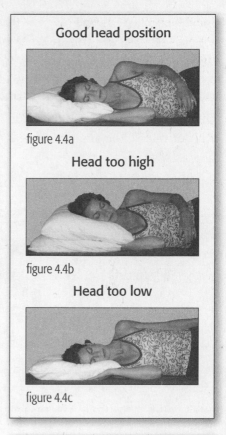

Good head position

figure 4.4a

Head too high

figure 4.4b

Head too low

figure 4.4c

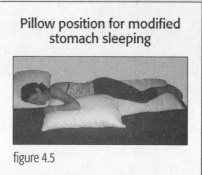

Pillow position for modified stomach sleeping

figure 4.5

Regardless of the task, your head's position and the strain on your neck and shoulder muscles will come into play. Often it is the times your mind is engaged in something else that you are least aware that what you are doing (or the way you are doing it) can be affecting your headaches. The eight common tasks below—four stationery, four moving—can serve as prime examples. If performed incorrectly, these tasks will place you in harm's way when it comes to your neck-based headaches. Pay close attention to the head-and-shoulder position changes suggested for each of them. They will be key players in getting you to the goal of headache relief.

1. Working at a Computer

The wrong setup:

- The computer monitor is too high, causing you to bend your head backward on your neck in order to view the screen.

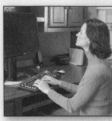
figure 4.6a

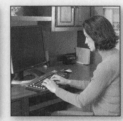
figure 4.6b

- Or, the computer monitor is too low, causing you to bend your head and neck forward and look down in order to view the screen.

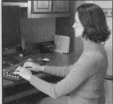
figure 4.6c

The right setup:

- When your head and neck are in proper alignment, the computer monitor is at eye level.

2. Working at a Desk or Table

The wrong setup:

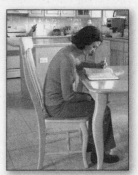

figure 4.7a

- You must hang your head forward and round your spine in order to read from or write on the work surface. (Our eyes seek to be at a 90-degree—perpendicular—angle to a work surface.)

The right setup:

- You're using a podium, wedge, or slant board to lift the work surface up to your eyes.*

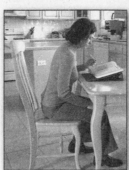

figure 4.7b

- You're using the hip-hinge method to lean toward the work surface to achieve the 90-degree angle your eyes seek. In other words, you're bending at the hips.

---

* A desktop/slantboard work surface can be purchased on my Web site, www.RestoringYourTemple.com.

3. Talking on the Phone

The wrong setup:

- You're cradling the phone between your ear and your shoulder while you work (even if your phone has a shoulder cradle attached to it).

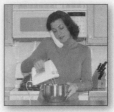

figure 4.8a

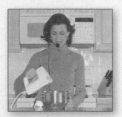

figure 4.8b

The right setup:

- Using a headset or the speaker phone feature on your phone. If your phone does not have these capabilities, make an investment in your health. Buy a phone that has one or both of these features and save yourself from a big pain in the neck!

4. Reading in Bed

The wrong setup:

- You're lying on your back with only your head and neck propped up on pillows. This sets up a right angle (90 degrees) between your neck and the rest of your body.

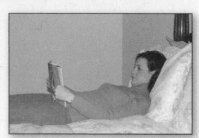

figure 4.9a

The right setup:

- Prop up your entire trunk with pillows against the headboard of your bed or the wall. This way a safe head and neck position can be maintained, and you can read all you want without compromising your neck.

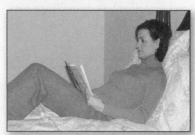

figure 4.9b

5. Carrying Briefcases and Pocketbooks

Directions:

1. If possible, use long straps on pocketbooks or briefcases and wear them across your body as shown in figure 4.10b. If you have one-sided neck pain, place the strap on the non-painful side.

2. Rethink your load. Can you use a waist pack rather than a handbag? Are you carrying around more than you need in your briefcase? Maybe you can use a backpack device (worn on *both* shoulders) rather than something that needs to be held onto with your overused upper trapezius muscle (see figures 3.1a and b).

Don't

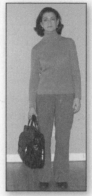

figure 4.10a

Do

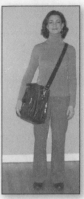

figure 4.10b

6. Lifting Loads Above Your Shoulders

Don't

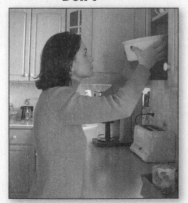

figure 4.11a

Do

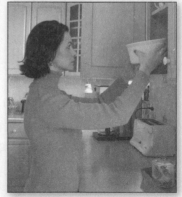

figure 4.11b

Directions:

1. Begin by facing your hips toward the load you're lifting.

2. Pinch your shoulder blades together in the down-and-back position for added strength and stability for your shoulders.

3. Lift the object (or objects) off its resting surface and, if need be, turn your feet (not your back) to face your hips toward the final destination of the load.

4. Lift the load above your shoulders (while exhaling for heart health), all the while maintaining safe and secure shoulder-blade and head and neck positioning.

---

7. Leaning Toward Work and Eating Surfaces

Don't   **Do**

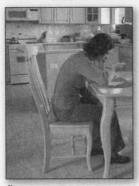   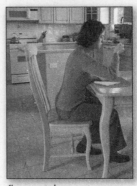

figure 4.12a   figure 4.12b

Directions:

1. When you need to lean forward over a desk or tabletop, use the hip-hinging method, rather than slumping your shoulders and flattening the backward curve *(lordosis)* of your low back.

2. Begin with good head, neck, and low-back posture.

3. Put your knees wider apart than your hips (to allow for freedom of movement from your hip joints) and bend forward by *bending from your hip joints.* If you slump forward from your spine, you

will "open up" the space where the front of your thigh meets your pelvis. If you perform this movement the correct way, your stomach will move *closer* to your thigh, narrowing the space between your trunk and thigh.

8. Applying Makeup or Shaving

Don't	**Do**
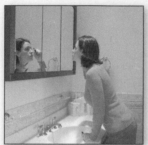	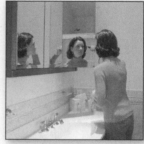
figure 4.13a	figure 4.13b

Directions:

1. Either move your entire body (from your feet up) closer to the mirror, or get a mirror on an extendable arm to use during grooming. This way you will not be jutting your chin forward (which is stressful to the discs and joints in your neck) while you work on your face.

2. With the exception of shaving your neck (men, I hope), you should avoid bending your head backward on your neck. Even when applying mascara (women, I hope), keep a safe and healthy head and neck posture working for you as you "ready yourself for public viewing."

Above all the other DIY treatment approaches you'll encounter in this book, postural corrections will have the greatest and most lasting impact on headache elimination. By making the changes recommended in this chapter, many of you will achieve a decrease in frequency or intensity of your headaches within the first 48 hours! And when you get to the point where your headaches are completely resolved, continued attention to proper posture will help you remain head-pain-free. I can't emphasize it enough: *good posture = pain relief.*

Chapter 5

Do-It-Yourself: Relief from Stiff Muscles, Stiff Joints, and Disc Pain

Tight muscles abound in the necks and chests of most headache sufferers. Whether you have neck-related headaches or classic migraines, the DIY stretching program in this chapter is for you.

Why is stretching so crucial? Well, tight muscles, having become shortened, no longer have the ability to be stretched to their full, natural length. Thus they create pain in a number of ways. First, their stiffness leads to pain every time their shortened length is challenged, such as when fully turning your head while driving or when looking down at the newspaper or a handheld device. Second, the increased tension in a tight neck or chest muscle presses on nearby nerves, causing pain to be referred to the head. Finally, a shortened muscle with trigger points loses a good deal of its strength, making it susceptible to overuse injury.

How did your muscles get so tight anyway? Well, poor posture, overloaded tasks, and brain-based pain can all lead to muscle dysfunction (tightening, increased tone, trigger points, or a combination of these). Good news. Regardless of the cause, you can quickly restore flexibility to your shortened neck and chest muscles. I have identified six key muscles that I find to be tight in nearly all of my headache patients. These muscles are either directly responsible for head pain, or they act as accomplices by preventing your body from getting into a healthy upright posture. Because dysfunction in these muscles is so widespread among headache sufferers, this stretching program "hat" will surely fit *your* "head."

Stretch-ology 101

Before you begin stretching, it is important we go over the "hows" of stretching. Here are those key points, in a mini-course I like to call "Stretch-ology 101."

- First of all, when you're lengthening a muscle, *the stretch intensity should be about a 5 on a scale of 1 to 10.* Not so much pulling that it feels painful, and not so little that it is quite comfortable. The muscle needs to feel like it is being stretched. If not, the brain will not get the "lengthen" message. On the other hand, if the stretch intensity is too great, instead of elongating, the muscle will instead contract and try to shorten. This occurs because it is trying to protect itself from a perceived threat (muscle tear) from the excessive stretching strain.

- Secondly, *each stretch should be held for a duration of 30 seconds.* The stretch needs to be a smooth, steady hold. No bouncing! There are two elements to a muscle: *elastic* and *plastic*. Bouncing is absorbed by the muscle's *elastic* element, much like pulling on a rubber band. This stretches the rubber band temporarily, but there is no lasting effect on its length.

  Muscles are truly lengthened only by affecting their *plastic* component. Did you ever play with a Slinky as a child? It came tightly coiled in its box from the store. Once you played with it for a while, invariably you would leave it hanging from something for too long a period of time. The result was, it never quite returned to its nicely coiled form. The Slinky's "plastic element," if you will, became permanently deformed (lengthened). In the body, the plastic element of our muscles is affected only when a lengthened muscle position (a stretch) is held over time, specifically 30 seconds of time.

Stretching the Six Key Muscles

Each muscle in the six key stretches for head pain is illustrated below with a drawing, so you'll know exactly where in your body you should feel the stretch as you perform it. If by chance you feel the stretch in a location *other* than the muscle region shown, try the stretch again with less force. If you continue to feel the stretch elsewhere, hold off and allow a health-care professional perform it for you.

1. Suboccipital Stretch

Back of head and neck

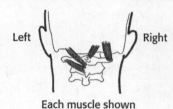

Left　　　　Right

Each muscle shown
is one of a pair.

figure 5.1

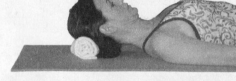

figure 5.2

Directions:

1. Make a firm, 3-inch-diameter towel roll out of a hand towel.

2. Lie on your back and place the towel roll under the lower portion of your skull. The correct location can be found by feeling along the back of your head just above your neck. You will find a prominent bony peak at the back of your skull. Place the towel roll at this level.

3. When your head is properly placed on the roll, your chin will tuck down toward your throat.

4. You should feel a stretch in the back of your upper neck just below the base of your skull.

5. Lie there for *10 minutes*—yes, a whole 10 minutes! (Why complain? You get to take a nap.) I always suggest my patients do this stretch before bed each night since they are already in the lying-down mood.

6. Because this is a 10-minute stretch, it needs to be done only once per day (although twice could speed the process along).

2. Upper Trapezius Stretch

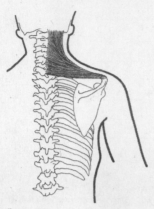

figure 5.3

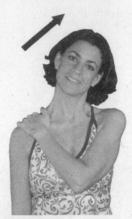

figure 5.4

Directions:

1. In a seated position, reach your left hand across your body and place it on top of your right shoulder.

2. Pull down on your right shoulder, depressing it. (I don't mean making it sad—simply lower it relative to your left shoulder.)

3. While maintaining the downward force on your right shoulder, slowly side-bend your head to the left, directing your left ear toward your left shoulder.

4. Stop when you feel a moderate stretch in the right side of your neck muscles.

5. Stretchology rules apply (see page 82).

6. Repeat three times on the other side if necessary.

3. Scalene Stretch

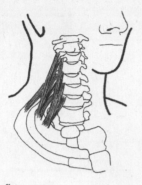

figure 5.5

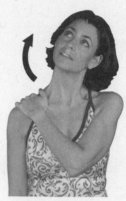

figure 5.6

Directions:

1. In a seated position, reach your left hand across your body and place it on top of your right shoulder.
2. Pull down on your right shoulder, depressing it (that is, lower it relative to your left shoulder).
3. While maintaining the downward force on your right shoulder, slowly side-bend your head to the left, directing your left ear toward your left shoulder.
4. Stop when you feel a mild stretch in the right side of your neck muscles.
5. Maintain this side-bending position while slowly rotating your face up toward the ceiling until you feel a moderate stretch in the front of your neck, on the right side.
6. Stretch-ology rules apply.
7. Repeat three times on the other side if necessary.

4. Sternocleidomastoid (SCM) Stretch

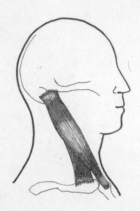

figure 5.7

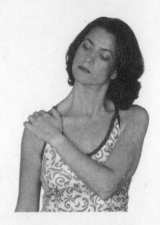

figure 5.8

Directions:

1. In a seated position, reach your left hand across your body and place it on top of your right shoulder.

2. Pull down on your right shoulder, depressing it (lower it relative to your left shoulder).

3. While maintaining the downward force on your right shoulder, slowly side-bend your head to the left, directing your left ear toward your left shoulder (as shown earlier in figure 5.4).

4. Stop when you feel a mild stretch in the right side of your neck muscles.

5. Maintain this side-bending position while slowly rotating your face up toward the ceiling until you feel a moderate stretch in the front of your neck, on the right side (as shown earlier in figure 5.6).

6. While maintaining this side-bent and rotated position, gently tuck your chin in toward your throat. You should feel a moderate stretch running from behind your right ear and extending down the right side of your neck.

7. Stretch-ology rules apply.

8. Repeat three times on the other side if necessary.

5. Levator Scapulae Stretch

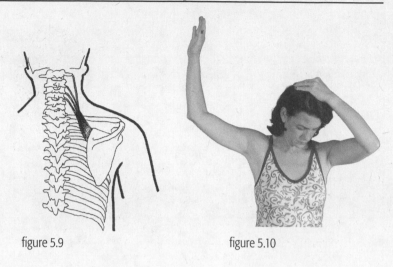

figure 5.9   figure 5.10

Directions:

1. Place a raised arm against a wall.

2. Turn your head away from your raised arm and slowly look down toward your opposite hip, tucking your chin into your throat as you lower your head.

3. Lightly place your other hand on top of your head and give a *gentle* overpressure to enhance the stretch.

4. Stop when you feel a moderate stretch in the right side of your upper back, running from your neck into the top of your shoulder blade.

5. VERY IMPORTANT: *Do not perform this exercise if you have a history of disc disease in your neck! Also, if pain is referred down into your mid-back or your arm, stop at once.*

6. Stretch-ology rules apply.

7. Repeat three times on the other side if necessary.

6. Pectoralis Major (Pec) Stretch

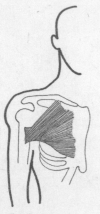

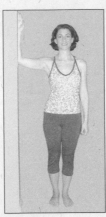

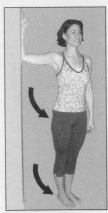

figure 5.11   figure 5.12a   figure 5.12b

Directions:

1. Stand next to a doorway or the outside corner of a wall.

2. Place your right forearm on the wall so your elbow is at the same height as your shoulder (see figures 5.12a and b). Your arm should be in line with your body, not in front or behind.

3. Turn your body to the left (away from the wall) by marching your feet in place to face off to the left. Allow the rest of your body to follow your feet. Don't overturn your neck to the left—your nose should stay in line with your breastbone.

4. Stop marching when you feel a stretch in your right front chest area.

5. Stretch-ology rules apply.

6. Repeat three times on the other side if necessary.

Fixing Bulged Discs While Loosening Stiff Joints

Living life with a forward-placed, backward-tipped "head block" can really stress out the discs in your neck. It also can make the joints in your neck so stiff that you will have a difficult time just trying to get into that good, upright posture we were talking about in chapter 4. If this is the case with you, these are two very effective exercises that can reduce disc bulging while freeing up your stiff neck joints. *Please use caution with these exercises if you have excessive neck pain and if you know you have herniated discs.*

Now, during these two exercises you may feel some increase in central neck pain (over your spine itself). However, any increase gained in central neck pain should stop immediately when you release the backward-gliding pressure. *You should never feel your pain travel outward across your shoulders or down your back or arms.* If either of these undesirable conditions occurs, try to lighten up on the pressure. And if that doesn't correct the situation, hold off on this exercise until you can put yourself in the hands of a professional.

---

1. Cervical Retraction on Pillow

Directions:

1. Lie on your back with one pillow under your head only (not under your shoulders).

2. Grasp your chin with both hands, with your elbows up off your chest as shown.

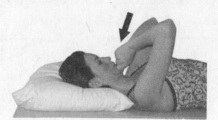

figure 5.13

3. Relax your neck muscles and slowly push your chin *backward* in the direction of the base of your skull as far as you can move it, and then release it slowly. (Avoid pushing your chin *down* into your throat so as to nod your head.)

4. Repeat for 3 sets of 10 repetitions, two to three times per day.

2. Cervical Retraction

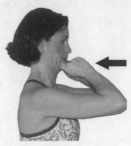

figure 5.14

Directions:

1. Sit up straight, with your hands grasping your chin as above and your elbows off your chest.

2. Slowly push straight back (not down), gliding your head back on your neck and your neck back over your shoulders.

3. Once you've pushed as far back as you can, don't hold your head in that position. Rather, release it slowly.

4. Repeat for 3 sets of 10 repetitions, two to three times per day.

When individual muscles, joints, or discs within your neck and chest areas become dysfunctional, pain is always just around the corner. For those of you reading this book, it already has come around the corner and hit you square on the head! That's why it's so important to work to restore normal length, motion, and structure to these components of your anatomy. You will be amazed at what these simple exercises can achieve in relieving your head pain. Be consistent, and you will most certainly be rewarded. Remember, no pain...all gain!

Chapter 6

Do-It-Yourself:
Core Strengthening
and Proper Breathing

Headaches resulting from muscle dysfunction often begin when your neck and shoulder-blade muscles are not up to the tasks they have to perform. Their weakness can develop over time or as a result of injury. Although there are many muscles surrounding your neck and shoulders, there are a special few that act as "internal stabilizers." They provide the underlying core strength and support necessary for your spine and all the other muscles in these two areas to function optimally.

As an analogy, consider the posts of a swinging gate. If they are properly secured in the ground, the gate will swing smoothly and latch consistently. Its hinges will have balanced forces on them and will not wear out prematurely. So it is for the joints, discs, muscles, and ligaments in your neck. You need your neck and shoulder-blade stabilizers to be in tip-top shape in order to secure (stabilize) your moving parts and prevent premature wear and tear on your joints, discs, and tendons. When these parts are not well-stabilized, muscle and joint dysfunction can result, which can then lead to pain referral to your head.

With that in mind, the following DIY muscle-strengthening exercises target four important muscle groups, two in the neck proper and two that help to control your shoulder blades. Without sufficient strength in these four groups, your body will have to call on other muscles in the area (the second-string players) to try to gain some stability. The one muscle that is always eager to volunteer for duty is the upper trapezius muscle. Remember how I showed you a stretch for him earlier (page 84)? The reason he is always tight is because he simply does too much work. But in his defense, if the first-string stabilizers are sitting on the bench, someone's got to play in the head-neck-shoulder game. So your goal here is to rehab the weakened first-string players so your upper trapezius can get back to playing his own position and not everyone else's.

Stabilizing Your Neck: The "LCs"

The first of the neck stabilizers we need to address is actually a pair of muscles: the *longus capitis* and *longus cervicis* (LCs for short, figure 6.1). Running down the front of the neck in close contact with your neck bones, the LCs have the very important job of giving rigidity to your neck. Upon initial contraction, they cinch the bones of your neck together, packaging them up as a unit. As they continue to contract and shorten, your head and neck are bent forward on your body. Your LCs are used every morning when you lift your head from your pillow and each time you bend your head forward to look down at something.

If your LCs are down for the count, larger muscles of your neck will take over. None of them have the intimate contact with the spine that the LCs do. They are physically unable to stabilize the individual bones. Therefore, whenever they act to lift your head or bend your neck forward, your unstabilized neck bones slide forward, unprotected, on each other, which creates significant shearing forces between the bones and discs (especially in your lower neck). Arthritic

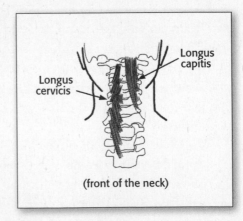

Longus capitis

Longus cervicis

(front of the neck)

figure 6.1

changes and disc degeneration are the results. This is why most herniated or bulging discs in the cervical spine occur in the *lower* neck (usually at the levels of C5 through C7). For this reason, we need to make sure the stable foundation of the LCs exists so we can build normal neck function upon it.

Longus Capitis and Longus Cervicis (LCs)
Exercise: Chin Tucks

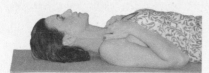
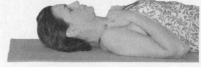

figure 6.2a   figure 6.2b

Directions:

1. Lie on your back with your head on a soft pillow.

2. Place your fingertips above your collar bone on the soft muscles of the lower throat area. You will be monitoring these muscles, making sure they don't contract during this exercise. If they do contract in an attempt to substitute for the longus cervicis, you will feel them become firm and ropy. (To feel this, gently lift your head from the pillow. See? The muscles tighten and swell under your fingers.)

3. Gently nod your head forward to look at your chest, and then relax your head back into the pillow. If the substitute muscles tighten up, try again—this time with a smaller movement of the head.

   I've had a number of patients who just couldn't get this at first. We would have to start with only their eyes glancing down toward their chests. But once they retrained their eye movements to occur without muscle substitution, we could add the head nod. If I'm describing you, once you reach this point, begin with tipping your nose downward just half a centimeter. As you are able to overcome the substitution, expand your range of nodding movement.

⟨RIGHT⟩

- The muscles you're monitoring are quiet.
- Your head remains resting on the pillow during the chin tuck.
- Fatigue is felt deep in the front of your neck.

⟫WRONG⟪

- Substitution with neck muscles being monitored by your fingers.
- Your shoulders move during the chin tuck.

Goal:

Continue until you are able to reach an endurance of 1½ to 2 minutes. Work up to this by performing the exercise 2x/day. Advance it by performing it in an upright position, either sitting or standing. This upright chin-tucking is an important daily task for the LCs. How many times do we look down throughout the day? We check our car's speedometer—well, maybe not all of us—we look down at what we're eating, we read the paper, we check our cell phones. I can't even type these words without looking down!

More Neck Stability: The "C-PVMs"

The second important muscle group to strengthen is your *cervical paravertebral* muscles. Those are big words, so let's break them down. *Cervical*, as you know by now, is another word for *neck. Para* means "alongside of," and *vertebral* refers to the vertebrae or spine. Thus these neck muscles run alongside your spine. For simplicity's sake we'll call them by their initials: the *C-PVMs*.

Your C-PVMs begin at the bottom of your skull and run down the back of your neck (as shown in figure 6.3). They are actually a group of three muscles that we use together for a single, important purpose. When they contract by themselves, they function to backward-bend your head and neck. However, when paired with the chin-tucking contraction of the LCs, the C-PVMs cause your head and neck to *glide,* or slide, backward together as a unit. This allows you to realign yourself and achieve proper head-on-neck and neck-on-shoulders posture.

The C-PVMs need to be restored to the stability game before we can invite the muscles of your shoulder-blade area to play. If we do not, we risk upsetting your neck while trying to strengthen your shoulder-blade muscles. Neck insults can lead to headaches—and that is the last thing we want!

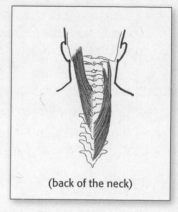

(back of the neck)

figure 6.3

Cervical Paravertebral Muscles (C-PVMs)
Exercise: Face-Lying Head Lifts with Chin Tuck

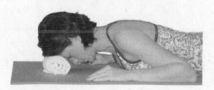

figure 6.4a

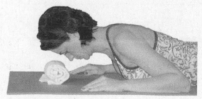

figure 6.4b

Directions:

1. Lie facedown, with your forehead on a small towel roll (figure 6.4a).
2. Chin tuck.
3. Gently tighten your abdominal muscles (draw your belly button in toward your spine) and continue to breathe.
4. Raise your forehead 1 to 2 inches from the towel roll, leading with

the back of your neck, *not* with the top of your head. Your eyes should still be looking down at the floor. Also, your shoulders should remain relaxed and unmoved. (This exercise is all about your neck. Shoulders are not welcome here.)

5. Hold this position for 5 seconds.
6. Slowly lower your head and relax the chin tuck.
7. Repeat until you experience signs of fatigue.

❰ RIGHT ❱

- Your head and neck are level with your back at the end range (top) of the lift.
- Your chin tuck is maintained.
- Fatigue is felt in the back of your neck.

≫WRONG≪

1. Your head is tipped backward, creating a backward bend in your neck.
2. Your shoulders rise up toward your ears during the lift.

Goal:
Continue until you are able to reach an endurance of 15 reps with good control. Work up to this by performing the exercise 2x/day.

Getting Your Shoulder Blades Stable: The "SA"

Now that your neck muscles are better controlled, we can move on to the shoulder-blade area. The first stabilizer we want to retrain here is the *serratus anterior* (SA) muscle group. Take a long look at figure 6.5. It is difficult to visualize the SA's position on the body because most of it lies hidden beneath your shoulder blade, and the part that isn't hidden is covered by other muscles and by your arm hanging at your side. Even in a bodybuilder, the only portion of the SA that can be observed readily is the muscle's edge, which is located along the side of the ribs halfway between the nipple line and the side of the body. (It is often referred to as a bodybuilder's "serration.")

The primary job of conditioned SA muscles is to hold your shoulder blades snugly against the back of your rib cage while you're standing and sitting and when you use your arms in an elevated position. If your SA is weak, your shoulder blades will stick out from your rib cage, a condition called "winging." The SA also works in concert with other shoulder-blade muscles to provide controlled rotation movement of the shoulder blade as you raise and lower your arm.

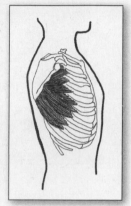

figure 6.5

Without controlled shoulder-blade stability, the upper trapezius muscle gets involved, and ultimately, tension is transferred to your neck. Problems in your neck send messages to your head and—voilà—you have a headache. Below you will find a beginning exercise, followed by a more advanced exercise. Once you've mastered the first (without shoulder-blade winging), move on to the second. There is no need to perform both exercises simultaneously.

Serratus Anterior (SA)
Exercise: Hands and Knees Rocking

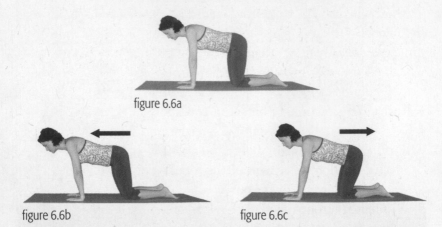

figure 6.6a

figure 6.6b   figure 6.6c

Directions:

1. Get in a crawling position, with your hands under your shoulders and your knees under your hips. Your knees should not be touching—rather, they should be about hip-width apart.

2. Gently tighten your abdominal muscles (draw your belly button in toward your spine) and continue to breathe.

3. Tuck your chin slightly (using the LCs we previously retrained) and draw your head up so it's about level with your neck, using your C-PVMs. (See why the treatment sequence is important?)

4. Push your rib cage gently up toward the ceiling until your shoulder blades are snugly seated against your back. (Remember not to lose your safe head and neck position.) If you have a second pair of eyes in your home—not belonging to a pet—you should ask them to watch your back to see if your shoulder blades are properly positioned. If you can't stop your shoulder blades from winging in this position, try the next exercise. You still may want to use that second pair of eyes, as the SA is the most difficult muscle to feel and monitor during retraining.

5. Once you are set up, rock about 1 inch forward and 1 inch backward over your hands. This challenges the SA to stabilize the

shoulder blade, mimicking weight-bearing activities such as washing a window, pushing open a door, pushing a shopping cart or baby stroller, and so on.

6. Once you've mastered this, try rocking side to side, again about 1 inch to the right and to the left.

7. For a real challenge, lift one hand off the floor and try to keep your shoulder blade from winging (no rocking here).

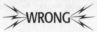

- Your shoulder blades stay in contact with the rib cage during the weight-shifting movements.
- Fatigue is typically not felt.

⋙WRONG⋘

- Your shoulder blades wing—lift off your back.
- You're unable to keep your neck in a safe, level position.

Goal:

Continue until you are able to reach an endurance of 20 reps. Work up to this by performing the exercise 2x/day.

Serratus Anterior (SA) Exercise: Wall Push-ups

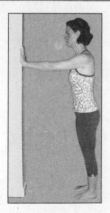 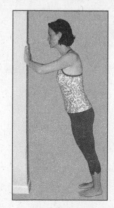

figure 6.7a   figure 6.7b

Directions:

1. Stand facing a wall, with your feet about 1½ to 2 feet from the wall surface.

2. Gently tighten your abdominal muscles (draw your belly button in toward your spine) and continue to breathe.

3. Lean forward, placing your hands on the wall at the height of your shoulders while keeping your elbows straight.

4. Push your rib cage gently backward until your shoulder blades are snugly seated against your back. (Remember to use the safe head and neck position described in the previous exercise.)

5. Begin bending your elbows, leaning forward toward the wall (just like in a floor push-up).

6. Push through your arms to return to a straight elbow position.

7. You may perform partial elbow bends if that is the only range in which you can control your shoulder blades. Work up to a full range. Challenge yourself by moving your feet further from the wall, increasing your body's incline.

◀ RIGHT ▶

- Abdominal contractions and your head and neck positions are maintained.
- Your shoulder blades are flush against your back throughout the exercise.
- Fatigue is not typically felt.

⚡WRONG⚡

- Your shoulder blades are winging.
- You're holding your breath.
- You're leading to the wall with your chin instead of your forehead.

Goal:

Continue until you are able to reach an endurance of 20 reps. Work up to this by performing the exercise 2x/day.

Keeping Your Shoulder Blades in Place: The "L-traps"

The *lower trapezius* (L-trap) muscle is the final stabilizer you'll need to strengthen. It performs a key role in posture by keeping your shoulder blades in a "down and back" position. If the L-trap isn't up to par, guess who jumps in the game again? That's right—the upper trapezius. Poor contraction of the L-trap causes the upper trapezius to pull relentlessly on your shoulder blades, dragging them upward so they sit higher up on your back.

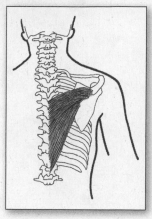

figure 6.8

The L-trap also plays a critical role in the upward rotation of your shoulder blade (a task it is supposed to share with your upper trapezius). Without sufficient L-trap strength, every time you reach upward to perform a task, instead of *rotating* upward, your shoulder blades are dragged farther up on your back by the unchallenged upper trapezius muscle.

In both cases, the upward gliding of your shoulder blades bunches up the muscles at the base of your neck, placing undue stress on all the local structures. And like I've indicated before, "If your neck muscles ain't happy, your head ain't gonna be happy either." Seriously, by strengthening your L-trap, you will restore muscle balance to your neck and shoulder-blade areas. In turn, muscle-tension headaches and trigger-point headaches will begin to disappear. Now that's worth working for!

Lower Trapezius (L-trap)
Exercise: Shoulder-Blade Retraction Glides

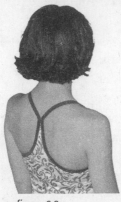
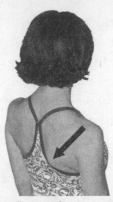

figure 6.9a   figure 6.9b

Directions:

1. Sit in a well-aligned posture, as demonstrated on page 71.

2. Gently place the fingertips of your left hand into the muscle on top of your right shoulder (the upper trap). With this hand you will be monitoring the upper trap muscle, making sure it does not contract. If it does, you will either feel your right shoulder lift up toward your ear, or you will feel the upper trap muscle become hard and swell under your fingertips. This is *bad.* We don't want any upper trap volunteerism!

3. Gently tighten your abdominal muscles (draw your belly button in toward your spine) and continue to breathe.

4. With your right arm at your side, hand resting in your lap, glide your right shoulder blade down and back (retraction)—as if you were directing it toward the back pocket of your pants.

5. Hold this position of retraction for 2 seconds.

6. Allow your shoulder blade to return slowly to its original position, and repeat the cycle until signs of fatigue set in.

7. Practice this glide until it is a smooth down-and-back motion without any interference from the volunteer!

8. Repeat the exercise on the other side.

9. When both sides are independently capable of performing the retraction movement, try them together. When the L-traps are used together, you will feel as if your neck is lengthening every time you retract your shoulder blades.

‹RIGHT›

- You feel a smooth gliding motion.
- Your trunk is not turning—only your shoulder blade is involved.
- Fatigue is felt in your mid-back area.

≫WRONG≪

- Your shoulder blade first moves either upward or toward the other shoulder blade before heading down and back toward your back pocket (poor coordination of movement).
- Your trunk turns toward the side of shoulder-blade movement.

Goal:
Continue until you are able to reach an endurance of 20 reps. Work up to this by performing the exercise 2x/day.

Lower Trapezius (L-trap)
Exercise: Arm Lifts from Ball

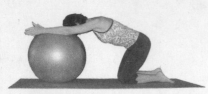

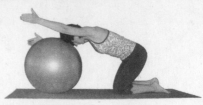

figure 6.10a   figure 6.10b

Directions:

1. Place a cushion on the seat of a chair and kneel down in front of it.*

2. Raise your arms over your head and lean forward, placing your forehead and your arms on the cushion (or ball) as shown.

3. Gently tighten your abdominal muscles (draw your belly button in toward your spine) and continue to breathe.

4. Lift one arm about 3 inches off the chair (or ball) and hold it there for 3 seconds.

5. Slowly lower it, and then repeat.

6. Continue lifting and lowering your arm until you feel signs of fatigue.

7. Repeat the exercise with your other arm.

◀ RIGHT ▶

- Your arm movements are smooth.
- Fatigue is felt in your mid-back area.

⚡WRONG⚡

- You're holding your breath.
- You're unable to maintain the gentle abdominal contraction.

Goal:

Continue until you are able to reach an endurance of 15 reps. Work up to this by performing the exercise 2x/day.

---

* Exercise balls like the one pictured above are available on my Web site, at www.RestoringYourTemple.com.

The Right Way to Breathe

"Okay, now you've gone too far, Lisa...Breathing? How can there be a right way and a wrong way to breathe? You just suck in and air fills your lungs, right?"

I'm sorry to burst your air bubble, but you may actually be breathing the wrong way. Faulty breathing patterns have been given the fancy name of *paroxysmal breathing*. More commonly this is known as *upper-chest breathing*. In upper-chest breathing, a person inhales by contracting the scalene muscles of their neck (see figure 5.5), which pull upward on their first and second rib attachments. The only time God meant us to use these muscles for inhaling is during activities that cause heavy, labored breathing. Otherwise, your scalenes were designed to be used exclusively for neck motion. If these muscles are overused for breathing (or otherwise), they will tighten and make your neck very unhappy. Say it with me this time: "If your neck ain't happy, your head ain't gonna be happy either!"

So what then is the right way to breathe? Humans were designed to draw in their breath by using their abdominal diaphragm, a process known as *diaphragmatic breathing*. The abdominal diaphragm is a dome-shaped muscle that attaches to your rib cage from front to back and side to side. Its presence separates your lungs and heart from your abdominal contents. When your diaphragm contracts, its dome flattens out and creates a vacuum in your chest cavity, which in turn causes air to be pulled into your lungs. When your diaphragm relaxes, the reverse happens, and air is pushed out of your lungs—exhalation.

Now, no one is born an upper-chest breather. (All babies breathe with their bellies—just watch 'em.) There are several reasons people *become* upper-chest breathers. Some are very concerned with their abundance of abdomen, if you know what I mean. In order to keep their tummies looking as minimal as possible, they suck in their stomachs or jam themselves into pants that are too tight at the waist. All this hinders their diaphragms from fully contracting. The only option they have is to breathe with their scalenes. Another reason for upper-chest breathing, one that especially plagues our society today, is stress and anxiety. When you or I become stressed out or anxious about something, we tend to take shallow, upper-chest breaths. As a result, we lose our natural, healthy diaphragmatic breathing pattern and replace it with neck-aggravating upper-chest breathing.

The best way to determine which way you breathe is to first lie on your back. Then place one hand on your tummy, just below your rib cage, and one hand over your breastbone. Now breathe normally, in and out, and feel which hand is moving. If you are an upper-chest breather, your "chest hand" will rise each time you breathe in. If you are breathing properly (diaphragmatically), your tummy hand will rise when you breathe in. (It is also normal if your chest rises *after* your tummy rises.)

If you find yourself guilty of scalene-muscle abuse (upper-chest breathing), you can give yourself a light sentence: Simply retrain yourself to relax your stomach and allow breathing to begin with your abdomen. I tell my patients to picture their stomach as a balloon they are filling up with each inhaled breath. Begin this in the back-lying position. Once you've got the hang of it, try it next while sitting and finally while standing.

Ice Can Be Your Friend

Whenever I get a neck-based headache that just won't quit, I reach for an ice pack. Not just any ice pack—rather, a soft gel pack covered with a wet paper towel. (Wet paper towels transfer the cold to your body much better than a wet—or dry—cloth towel.) I place this ice pack at the junction between the back of my head and the top of my neck, right along my hairline.

Sometimes 10 minutes in this position is all you'll need for relief. If the headache is a really bad one, you may need to remain on that ice up to 45 minutes. This is not excessive, because the cold of the ice is being transferred through the buffer of your hair. If you use the ice pack directly against your skin, such as lower on your neck or across your forehead, then 10 minutes is enough. (You don't want to get bit by Jack Frost.) I have my patients begin with the ice at the base of their heads, as above, but I tell them to then move it to wherever they feel it may help.

Why ice—when most people tell you to wrap a moist heating pad around your shoulders? Because headaches are inflammatory in nature. Muscles are in acute, painful spasm, and blood vessels and nerves are swollen. Cold is an anti-inflammatory agent. Heat is just the opposite. It brings blood to the area, further congesting the muscles and swelling the blood vessels. If the headache medicine you reach for is an anti-inflammatory (Advil, Aleve, Motrin) it makes sense that you would want to use an anti-inflammatory agent—ice—locally as well. The second great thing about ice is, it's antispasmodic, meaning it breaks up muscle spasms. Two great benefits from one ice pack—that's sure to send a chill up your spine!

The End...of Your Headaches?

As you add the DIY treatment approaches in chapters 4 through 6 to your daily life, you will almost certainly notice marked changes in your headaches. Chronic headaches don't disappear in a day, or even a week. Rather, headache resolution tends to follow a pattern:

1. Typically, headaches change by first becoming *less intense.*
2. Then, your headaches last for a *shorter period of time.*
3. Next, you'll experience *greater headache-free time* between your head-pain episodes.
4. Finally, *your headaches will fade away.* A new day will have dawned for you. Hallelujah, no more head pain!

While these changes are in the making, be *patient* and *diligent.* The better you reform your ways, lengthen and strengthen your muscles, and protect yourself against harmful postures, the better and faster your outcome will be.

My hope is that you are able to overcome your headaches on your own. However, if you've applied all that you now know to do and are still left with a portion of your headache, read on through the next chapter. There I provide advice on who to seek hands-on treatment from and what to expect from their treatment approaches.

Chapter 7

Putting Yourself in the Hands of a Professional

When you take an overall view, tension-type headaches and cervicogenic headaches can stem from many of the same issues: upper neck-joint dysfunction; disc problems; and muscular conditions such as trigger points, spasms, tightness, and weakness. All of these, in one way or another, "get on your nerves" and send pain complaints into your head. And you know what the end result is...a terrible headache.

Many people reading this book will be able to fully relieve their own neck-based or neck triggered headaches simply by applying the DIY recommendations I gave in the last three chapters. Maybe your hopes are up because you have diligently followed my advice and have found significant relief from your head pain. Although you know you're on the right track, your final headache-free destination somehow eludes you. Or you may be one of those occasional sufferers whose headaches are so awful and so chronic that no matter what you try, your head pain refuses to budge.

If you fall into one of these last two groups and have not been able to get *full* relief on your own, then your next step in the headache-elimination process is to find a hands-on professional who is well qualified to both evaluate and treat your condition. Now, I reckon that if you knew just who this hands-on, headache-treating professional was, you'd have gone to 'em a long time ago! So allow me to give you some counsel.

First, I believe all headache care should begin with conservative, hands-on treatment. Only if conservative treatment fails to bring about successful results should you then seek more invasive procedures. For neck-related headache treatment, invasive procedures are injections on the lower end of the spectrum and neck surgery on the high end. I have never personally known a patient whose only complaint was headaches to end up at the surgeon's office. However, there are infrequent occasions when people with severe neck pain coupled with headaches will not respond to noninvasive or low-level invasive procedures (injections). These people will ultimately need to undergo surgery to find relief.

All Hands on Deck

There are three fields of traditional health care that treat headache patients using a hands-on approach. They are *physical therapy, chiropractic,* and *massage therapy.* What do I mean by "hands-on" approach? It is just as it sounds (only better, since even a fistfight could qualify as a hands-on approach!). Professionals in each of these disciplines have been trained to evaluate and treat patients with their "raw hands."

Depending upon their line of training, they may be able to tell if a joint, disc, or muscle is the root of the problem. Once a diagnosis of the problem has been made, such a practitioner can then treat someone using their very own hands! During these treatments they may move, mobilize, or manipulate a person's muscles or joints, and even possibly prescribe exercises to fix bulging discs.

Now, there is something you need to keep in mind. The three health disciplines I discuss in this chapter are not interchangeable. Each profession has different areas of trained expertise. (And remember, within each field, not all practitioners are created equal.) For those of you who may not be as familiar with these fields as you wish, in the following pages I explain their areas of specialty and their preferred treatment techniques and methods.

Physical Therapy

Physical therapy is a rehabilitation specialty that includes many subspecialties, such as orthopedics, neurology, pediatrics, cardiology, and others. Treatment settings vary from hospital-based to private practice, school settings, and even home care. Physical therapists (PTs) treat the muscles, nerves, joints, and discs of their patients' bodies with *exercises, hands-on techniques, modalities (moist heat, ice, ultrasound, electric stimulation, and others),* and *movement re-education.*

Presently, physical therapists' education requires a four-year undergraduate degree followed by completion of either a two-year masters or a three-year physical-therapy doctorate program. Students of the latter program graduate with a doctorate in physical therapy (a DPT) and may introduce themselves to their patients as "Dr. Such-and-such." However, their training should not be confused with that of a medical doctor (an MD)—it is totally different.

What to Look For

When looking for a physical therapist who is qualified to treat your headaches you should ask a prospective PT if he or she refers to themselves as a "manual physical therapist." This subgroup of physical therapists have taken extra training courses beyond their formal education, which focus on the evaluation and treatment of the spine, head, and jaw areas.

It is not unreasonable for you to ask if you can visit the physical-therapy facility and speak to the PT who will be treating you. (You can even bring this book along with you!)

- You will want to ask if they indeed practice manual physical therapy at their facility. Often a good rule of thumb for determining if you'll get adequate hands-on time is to ask about the facility's scheduling time frame. Are people scheduled every half hour or every 15 minutes? Practices that schedule less frequently are more apt to perform manual therapy treatment.

- Another question is, Will you see the same physical therapist (or at most two) each time you are treated, or is it a "free for all" in assigning therapists to patients? Treatment continuity declines the more hands you have treating you.

- Some PT practices "treat" their patients with semisupervised exercise programs, heat, and electric stimulation, but rarely if ever put their hands on them. If and when they do, it is for a general sort of relaxation massage, not accurate enough to bring about any lasting change.

• Talk to your prospective PT about their treatment approach for headache recovery. Does it include words or phrases such as *upper cervical spine, joint mobilization, trigger point release,* muscle *stretching* and *strengthening, postural re-education,* and *activities of daily living (ADL) retraining?* If so, sign up! It sounds like you'll be in good hands.

A manual physical therapist who is on the ball regarding headaches will treat your neck with

• *massage,* which will address trigger points, muscle tightness, spasm, or a combination of these three in your head, face and neck, and so on

• *muscle stretching*

• *safe joint-mobilization techniques* that specifically address

1. the right and left *occipito-atlantal (O-A) joints* (between the skull and the first neck bone),

2. the *atlanto-axial (A-A) joint* (between the first and second neck bones),

3. the position of the *atlas*—the first vertebra of the neck— itself (is it centered or off to one side?)

4. the right and left *C2-C3 facet joints* (You can visually refresh your memory of these joints back in chapter 3, figure 3.6.)

• …and basically *everything else I taught you in the last three chapters.*

Manual physical therapy is by far the most eclectic in its treatment approach, since it addresses all the possible mechanical components of headache production. The next two professions I discuss are more focused. But the problem with this can be that they have fewer chances of successfully hitting the headache-source "target."

A Technique I Recommend Avoiding

The upper neck joints, in my opinion, should never be treated with high-velocity manipulation or thrusting techniques ("joint cracking"). There have been documented cases—one most recently in Canada—where patients have suffered stroke and even death from this procedure. In 2002, Dr. Edzard Ernst, a British researcher, surveyed neurologists in Britain about cases of serious neurological complications occurring within 24 hours of manipulation of the cervical spine (MCS) by various types of practitioners.[1] After analyzing the results, he concluded,

> Clinicians might tell their patients to adopt a cautious approach and avoid the type of spinal manipulation for which the risk seems greatest: *forceful manipulation of the upper spine with a rotational element.* [2]

In a 1999 article in *Physical Therapy* magazine, researcher Richard DiFabio analyzed 177 cases that had been reported between 1925 and 1997.[3] He noted,

> Although the risk of injury associated with MCS appears to be small, this type of therapy has the potential to expose patients to vertebral artery damage that can be avoided with the use of mobilization (nonthrust passive movements).[4]

The injuries most frequently mentioned in the medical literature were *arterial dissection,* a tear in an artery's wall; *arterial spasm,* a constriction of the artery caused by a contraction of the smooth muscle in the wall of the artery; and *brain stem lesions,* disruptions of blood flow within the lower part of your brain.[5] All of these injuries can lead to stroke or death.

However, DiFabio also had some good news. He went on to say that "physical therapists were involved in less than 2% of the cases, and no deaths have been attributed to MCS provided by physical therapists."[6]*

The only reason I'm "getting scientific on you" is because I want to make a point. *High-velocity manipulation of the upper neck comes with a risk.* And I'd rather you *not* proceed at your own risk!

---

* Unfortunately, 60 to 70 percent of the injuries or deaths occurred at the hands of chiropractors.[7] Their method of treatment is primarily joint thrusting of a rotational nature.

Chiropractic

The field of chiropractic bases treatment of physical illness and pain on the *alignment* of one's spine. Most chiropractors work in a private practice setting. The method by which they *align* their patients' spines is primarily high-velocity joint manipulation (joint "cracking"). When a spinal joint is manipulated in this fashion, typically an audible "crack" will be heard, followed by immediate (but often short-lived) muscle-tension relief.

Chiropractic education consists of the completion of a four-year chiropractic program, which is preceded by at least two years of undergraduate study in basic sciences. Upon graduating, chiropractors, like their PT counterparts, may introduce themselves to their patients as "Dr. Such-and-such." Again, this is not to be confused with a medical doctor (MD). Often, a medical doctor will list their name and credentials as, for example, "William Smith, MD," while a chiropractor will typically use, for example, "Dr. William Smith," and then list the title "Chiropractor" underneath. (This is important to understand, because some people fail to get regular checkups from their medical doctors because they are regularly treated by their chiropractor.)

Over the past 15 to 20 years, the field of chiropractic has expanded the scope of its practice to include the use of traditional physical therapy modalities such as ultrasound and electric stimulation as well as offering massage therapy as a supplement to chiropractic care. In the Northeast United States, for example, chiropractic facilities also offer general health and wellness training, nutritional supplements, and sometimes even tai chi classes.

What to Consider

The primary method used by most chiropractors when treating head and neck pain is, again, high-velocity manipulation of the neck joints. (See sidebar on the risk when these thrusts are performed in the upper neck.) Joint manipulation has its place, but I believe it is often overused.

Many years ago, while taking a step class at the gym, I noticed a woman in the back of the room who was performing the exercises without using her arms. I immediately thought she must be avoiding neck or shoulder pain. When the class was over, I (very uncharacteristically for me) told her I'd noticed she wasn't using her arms in class and wondered if she had neck pain.

She told me that not only did she have neck pain, but right arm pain as well. She told me she couldn't even lift her right arm enough to reach for her purse on the passenger's seat in the car. "Have you had any treatment?" I asked. "Yes, I go to the chiropractor. I've been going for six years." I'm sure my mouth dropped open. That was more than enough treatment under anyone's care.

"I'm not guaranteeing anything," I began, "but I'm a physical therapist and I specialize in treatment of the spine. If you'd like to try a new approach, I believe I can help you. I've never treated anyone for longer than six months." Well, in short, this woman came to my office, and I found that her neck joints were so loose and mobile, it was scary. She had been overmanipulated. Her upper back joints, her right rib cage, and the nerves running down her right arm all had issues that had never been addressed. When these areas were treated using manual physical therapy techniques, this woman regained full use of her arm and was pain-free within five months. "Everything in moderation" makes sense, even when referring to joint manipulation.

There are patients who receive headache help in the hands of chiropractors. Again, word of mouth is a good way to find a good set of chiropractic hands. It is still my opinion that the upper neck should not be thrusted ("cracked"), given the incidents of injury that have, on rare occasions, resulted. I wouldn't want you to take that chance. Discuss this with your chiropractor during your evaluation. You can certainly ask him or her not to use high-velocity manipulation in your upper neck.

Spinal Terminology

Long ago the field of chiropractic care coined the terms *slipped disc* and *subluxation*, which have made their way into today's common language. Both of those terms, while catchy, don't reflect the true structure of the body. Discs don't "slip," and spinal joints don't "sublux" readily. What does happen is that discs *bulge* or *herniate* and spinal joints *lose motion* (become stiff) in a particular direction. (*Subluxation,* correctly used, refers to a bone that slips beyond its normal range of motion—"out of joint"—momentarily and then slips back into proper alignment.)

Massage Therapy

Massage therapists used to be called by the French terms *masseuses* (female) or *masseurs* (male). They typically work in private-care settings and may even do house calls. The length of their massage-therapy schooling will depend on which program is attended, but it usually lasts between six months and two years. Massage therapists are trained in various treatment techniques that affect the length, tension, and tone of muscles by way of *hands-on soft-tissue mobilization* (massage).

While there are different types of massage, the one thing they all have in common is the use of the hands (manual technique) and the mobilization of muscles. Massage forms include shiatsu, Rolfing, Swedish massage, deep-tissue massage, and many others. Some alternative forms of massage therapy include "off the body" techniques, which purport to redirect energy flow within the body and which have their origin in Eastern religion. (I personally do not recommend them for my own religious reasons.)

Massage therapists, typically, are not trained to evaluate overall posture, spinal joints, or anything beyond the muscles (strengthening not included). However, if your headaches are due purely to muscular dysfunction (trigger points, spasms), then you may do very well under the care of a massage therapist.

In conclusion, if you have tried one of these disciplines without success, do try the others before abandoning noninvasive treatment options for your head and neck. Also, if you have already tried one of these professionals, such as a PT, and after reading my description of "what to look for" have discovered you didn't get the best headache treatment, don't give up hope on the entire field of physical therapy. Try another practitioner.* This time you'll be more prepared for your search. If, however, you've exhausted your noninvasive neck-based-headache treatment options, then you will have to explore the more aggressive—invasive—approaches.

Physicians and Injections

Rarely does anyone look forward to someone sticking them with a needle. Memories of childhood vaccinations, blood work, and the like flood the mind at the mere thought of it. Not so with chronic head-pain sufferers. They have usually been around the health-care block—seen more specialists than they care to remember, taken a load of pills, undergone plenty of tests, followed everyone's advice—and still their pain remains. If this speaks of your experience, you will attest to the fact that you wouldn't care if someone stuck you with a needle or multiple needles at this point. You'll endure just about any-thing as long as there is hope that your suffering will be relieved.

The two fields of doctors who typically administer these injections are 1) medical doctors, specifically *neurologists, anesthesiologists,* and *pain-management specialists;* and 2) *dentists:* doctors of dental surgery (DDS) or doctors of medical dentistry (DMD). Look for a specialist who regularly treats head pain.

What Medications Are Used?

What kind of potentially pain-relieving injection am I talking about? Typically, they will contain a medicine called *lidocaine,* which acts on the body to numb pain. Lidocaine is an anesthetic, so it kind of puts your pain to sleep. Often, the lidocaine is mixed with another medicine called *hydrocortisone.* Hydrocortisone is a steroidal anti-inflammatory, meaning it reduces swelling (inflammation). By reducing local inflammation, this steroid "deflates" the angry, swollen nerves, blood vessels, joint capsules, and muscles that may be sending

---

* Visit my Web site, www.RestoringYourTemple.com. I provide more information on the page "Finding a Good PT."

your brain "headache telegrams." (You needn't be concerned about the "steroid" part. This type of steroid will not pump you up like a bodybuilder.)

Together these two medicines act to reduce or eliminate pain by both stopping the pain messages from traveling to your brain (lidocaine) and by stopping the pain messages from being "written" in the first place (hydrocortisone). Other "close cousins" of these two medicines may be used instead, but they will have the same effect. Unfortunately, many people experience head-pain relapse within three months. But even though these injections may need to be repeated cyclically, three months without a headache is a wonderful thing!

Another injection that has recently come into treatment vogue is *Botox.* Yes—the same Botox that has swept through Hollywood and is now being used to wipe away wrinkles from faces across the country. Botox is actually a weakened form of *bo*tulinum *tox*in, which is one of the most poisonous naturally occurring substances in the world! Though it is highly toxic, it is used in minute doses to treat not only unwanted wrinkles but painful muscle spasms and trigger points as well.

When Botox is injected, it essentially prevents the local nerves from sending their "contraction messages" to the surrounding muscle. The resulting effect is a paralyzed muscle segment. This is the best form of relaxation available, though extreme. Botox has been used effectively to achieve relief from head and neck pain. Problem is, it also is short-lived: about three months or so. Then another round of injections is needed.

Where Are the Medications Administered?

Injections meant to treat headaches are administered to different structures in the head and neck. The most common is the *intramuscular injection.* Muscles of the neck, head, or face are palpated (felt) for specific trigger points or areas of painful spasm. These areas of muscle dysfunction then become the target sites for injection. Both the lidocaine/hydrocortisone and the Botox injections are used this way.

Injections of lidocaine, hydrocortisone, or most likely a combination of the two can also be administered directly into the facet joints—joints between the vertebrae—of the neck. *Facet injections* can be especially useful in headache relief if performed at the C2-C3 facet level, as spoken about earlier. That said, it is quite possible for other painful facet levels in the neck to be adding to the overall tension in the neck muscles. Injecting these facets also may well provide added benefit.

Nerve blocks are another type of injection procedure. In these cases a "cocktail" of lidocaine and hydrocortisone (or similar drug cocktail) is injected with a specific spinal nerve as its target, usually the C2 or C3 spinal nerves. The effect on the spinal nerve is the same as with muscle injections: the numbing and decreasing of the swelling of the irritated nerve. Once again, the "last-ability" of this injection is three months or so.

Unfortunately, no type of injection is a sure thing for relieving headaches. While many people are helped, many others have unsuccessful outcomes. My rule of thumb is to try the least invasive methods of treatment first, as there is always a risk when you enter into the body, whether by oral or injected medication or by surgical intervention.

The Search for Good Hands

The world is full of restaurants. Some are fast-food, some try to be gourmet but fail the taste test, and some are truly spectacular. If the outside of the restaurant or the inside décor were consistently representative of the quality of the food, choosing a place to eat would be a piece of cake. This, however, is not always the case. My husband loves a good "hole in the wall" eatery. He has said countless times before that little mom-and-pop restaurants often serve the yummiest food. Many times he's been right.

So it is with physical therapy facilities and other medical offices. The proof is in the results. And, as with good restaurants, word of mouth is one of the best ways to find a pair of "good hands." Someone is vouching for their personal recovery experience. In the previous four chapters I have given you a "restaurant review" and informed you of the "secret recipe" for high-quality treatment of neck-related headaches. Choose wisely, and may your journey come out well!

And if you've been wondering how the "search for good hands" turned out for the two people with neck-based headaches (see chapter 3), I'd like to share the rest of their stories.

W.J.'s Tension-Type Headache Story

(Recap from chapter 3): He (my doctor) reluctantly gave me a prescription for physical therapy when I asked for it, but didn't seem confident it would help any. Boy was he wrong!

(Conclusion): I began physical-therapy treatment in January of 2004. I must say I was very skeptical, but I desperately needed some relief. My ability to function in any activity, for any length of time, was severely limited. My ability to enjoy any activity was minimal. I was in pain constantly, exhausted, and fearful I would have to live this way the rest of my life.

My physical therapy visits consisted of moist heat, electric stimulation, massage, gentle manual joint and disc mobilization, and exercises. Gradually, I began to feel better. After a few months my nagging headaches were gone, and my neck pain was tolerable. I faithfully did the home exercises my physical therapist taught me. Six months later I was feeling great!

It is now 2007 as I write this. I haven't had a single headache since completing my physical-therapy treatment in 2004 (unless I have a cold or virus). My neck will sometimes feel slightly stressed, especially after sitting at the computer or driving long distances, but the exercises always relieve my discomfort.

Today, I am an energetic, highly functioning, incredibly busy wife, mother, and grandmother. I am so thankful to be able to fully enjoy all that God has given me.

—W.J.

R.W.'s Cervicogenic Headache Story

(Recap from chapter 3): One day a friend suggested I try physical therapy. I was unsure of what a physical therapist would be able to do, but at this point, I was willing to try anything!

(Conclusion): During my first physical therapy evaluation I was made aware of my posture and how my particular neck and shoulder position related to my headaches. It wasn't good. My chest muscles were pulling my shoulders in, and my neck was leaning forward, pulling my shoulders up as if I was constantly shrugging them. I began treatment twice a week, which consisted of muscle massages, joint mobilization, muscle stretching, and home exercises.

Little by little, I began feeling the tension in my neck and shoulders lessen. I was starting to feel normal again. My headaches continued for a couple of weeks after beginning treatment, but they weren't as strong and they did not last for days at a time. After ten visits I had responded so well that I only need to be treated once a week.

Understanding how my body works and the importance of keeping my muscles stretched and elongated has helped me keep my head and shoulders in the proper, upright position. I am excited to say that (at the time of writing this) I have been headache-free for 32 days. Praise God. I am continuing weekly treatment for my remaining eye and cheek pain with confidence that these symptoms will soon be a thing of the past as well.

—R.W.

These two patients have seen what a good educator with a skilled pair of hands can do for a chronic headache situation. It is my prayer that you find equally good care for yourself. And that one day, you too will be headache-free.

Part 3

Brain Pain

Chapter 8

Migraines and Cluster-type Headaches

If you suffer with either migraine or cluster-type headaches, you have a lot of company. Today in the United States there are about 33 million migraineurs and roughly 1 million people who suffer with cluster-type headaches. While migraine headaches affect more women than men (3 to 1, or 75 percent), cluster headaches are almost exclusively experienced by men (9 to 1, or 90 percent).

If you are included in these statistics, you know that you typically manage your pain in social isolation. You must check out of the world around you while your head pain rages, and then check back in after the storm has passed. Many times your casual acquaintances and even some of your good friends won't know you suffer from these life-altering headaches—because, in between attacks, you seem perfectly well. And during the attacks...well, you're not in a socializing mood.

According to the latest scientific research, the feature that sets migraine and cluster headaches apart from the categories we've discussed earlier in this book is that these two appear to have their origin within the brain itself. These headaches—which do not appear to be caused by sources or referred pain—are truly *brain pain*.

Now, the brain itself is not a pain-sensitive structure, therefore it cannot "hurt." This is why brain surgery can be performed on someone who is fully awake. On the other hand, the brain does control the release and blocking of certain chemicals that affect the nerves and blood vessels surrounding it. It is these nerves and blood vessels that are pain-sensitive and which therefore can become head-pain-producing.

Although it is correct to say that the *why* of these headaches is not fully understood, science is getting a clearer picture as to the *what, when,* and *where.* Many important puzzle pieces have been discovered in recent years, which have been illuminating our understanding of the headache process. Originally, scientists believed headaches were caused by too much blood flow in the brain and head. Next, researchers shifted to blaming inflamed nerve endings within the head. Currently, the *neurogenic theory* has replaced both of these earlier ideas. It proposes that the headache process is initially driven by chemical reactions occurring within the brain itself, which first affect the nerves and eventually the surrounding blood vessels.

Are Migraine Sufferers Just Thick-Headed?

According to the research of Dr. Nouchine Hadjikhani, published in 2007 in the medical journal *Neurology,* the answer is *yes.* When Dr. Hadjikhani and her colleagues compared the brain MRIs of 24 people who suffered from migraines with 12 people who did not, they found that the *somatocortex* (the outer sensory portion of the brain) was on average *21 percent thicker* in those who suffered with migraines. Even more notable was that this thickening was most significant in the area where sensations from the trigeminal area, the head, and the face are processed (see chapter 1).

Is this thickening of the brain's cortex the contributing factor to migraines, or does having repeated migraines cause this area of the brain to thicken? Excellent question—and unfortunately, we'll have to wait for future studies to determine the answer.

The Known Facts of Brain Pain

As of 2007, the best brain-pain theory begins with the known fact that the brains of migraine and cluster-headache sufferers are different from the brains of those who experience occasional headaches. While more is presently known about migraines than about cluster headaches, science continues to uncover further information leading to a clearer understanding of the source of both. The greater our knowledge base is, the better our intervention. Many of the methods and medications we use today stem from the recent revisions in our understanding of cause and effect.

Scientific research has established the following five facts about migraine pain and its associated symptoms:

1. *Migraineurs are overstimulated by what they see and hear.* Their brains are hypersensitive to both visual and auditory stimulation. For example, migraine sufferers can see flashes of light at a much lower power-pulse than nonmigraineurs. Secondly, their brains are not able to get used to repetitive visual or auditory stimulation in the same way the brains of their non-headache counterparts are. Therefore, rather than being able to ignore annoying sight and sound inputs, their brains "dwell on them," so to speak.

2. *Pain starts deep within the brain.* There is at least one area within the brain that initiates and maintains the migraine process. The best identified source is located in the brain stem. (The brain stem sits under the main part of the brain, close to the spinal cord in the upper neck.) Scientists have nicknamed this "overactive" area the *migraine generator.* It has been shown to receive incoming emotional and pain messages from the mind and body (such as "my teen is making my life insane" or "my neck is killing me") and respond with an outgoing pain reply ("Let's throw a brain-pain dinner party. We'll begin with an inflammatory appetizer, serve up a main course of throbbing with a side of nausea, and finally end with some physical exhaustion for dessert!").

3. *Vision changes are caused by an electrically charged wave washing over the brain.* Visual *auras* (flashing light, altered vision) are the result of increased electrical activity sweeping across the brain's surface, followed by a wave of decreased electrical charge. Accompanying these electrical changes is a brief period of increased brain blood flow, followed by a

drop in blood flow. The bright lights seen by a migraineur are the result of the initial increase in electrical brain activity, and the *visual loss* (dark, gray, or white opaque areas) is the result of the subsequent drop in electrical activity.

4. *A swollen "brain" equals throbbing pain.* The throbbing pain of a migraine is caused by inflammation (swelling) of the brain's surface blood vessels and the brain's covering (the *meninges*). As a result of the electrical changes above, the nerve endings of a migraineur's brain release inflammatory proteins that cause the small blood vessels they come into contact with to enlarge and leak. This leakage aggravates the nerve endings of the surrounding blood vessels and brain covering, ultimately giving rise to throbbing head pain.

5. *Too painful to touch.* Migraine sufferers often develop *allodynia*—a sensitivity to normally nonpainful physical touch. This hypersensitivity affects the migraineur's scalp, head, or neck area, or a combination. Sometimes it extends as far down as the arm. So if your hair hurts when you have a migraine, or if you are sensitive to breezes or clothing and jewelry around your neck, you are not crazy—nor are you alone in experiencing this phenomenon. This common symptom typically sets itself in motion one to four hours into your migraine. Once it is in progress, however, aborting your headache will be more difficult. So take your migraine-abortive medication before its onslaught.

I love to see it when science explains life's mysteries. It always points me to how fearfully and wonderfully we have been created. What a miracle it is that our bodies function the way they do, with such precision—and how devastating are the results when something seemingly small—in the brain, for example—malfunctions.

The Dark Days of Migraines

Only a migraineur can describe his or her particular headache. While there are definite common characteristics, an individual's migraine experience can be as unique as their own signature. I want you to see what is common and what is unusual in migraine experiences. If you've truly been experiencing migraines, I hope you will be able to see yourself, at least partially, in one of the following stories—and that you will find comfort in knowing you are not alone and you are certainly not crazy!

Briefly—since details were already given in chapter 1—there are four distinct phases of migraine. (However, not all four need to be experienced in order for a person to be classified as a migraineur.) The first is called *prodrome*. During this phase, a person may experience sensitivity to light, sound, or smells; stiffness in their neck; feelings of fatigue or anxiety; food cravings; and other "odd sensations." These sensations or sensitivities can occur anywhere from a few hours to a few days before a headache begins.

The second phase, the *aura*, lasts, on average, less than 60 minutes. In most cases, it directly precedes head pain. Typical factors experienced during this phase include visual disturbances; light and noise sensitivity; nausea, vomiting, or both. Less common aura symptoms can include tingling (pins and needles) in the head, arms, or face; smelling odors that are not present; difficulty speaking; and one-sided muscle weakness. Though nausea and vomiting during the headache phase are quite common (70 percent and 50 percent of the time, respectively), auras preceding head pain are experienced by only 20 percent of migraineurs. With that in mind, here's the story of a former patient of mine who was one of that unfortunate 20 percent.

Migraine with Prodrome and Aura

When I was nine years old, I was struck by a jet skier while water-tubing on a family vacation. I suffered a fractured right collarbone and had multiple small fractures on the right side of my skull. A year or so following my injuries, my neck muscles on the right side would periodically become tight and I would have to crack my neck in order to get some relief. Unfortunately, shortly following this neck tightness, I would feel a migraine coming on.

In actuality, I would have an even earlier sign. Two to three days before a migraine, I would have frequent episodes of déjà vu. Suddenly, I would feel as if I had been in that same place-in-time before, looking at the same things, and hearing the same voices. (I know that may be a little weird for most people to understand.) Following this, I would begin to feel dizzy, my insides would get shaky, and my head would begin to hurt. The weird symptoms would last about 30 seconds and then pass.

Like clockwork, two to three days later I would wake up in the morning primed for a migraine. I would start out with having those strange feelings I'd had in the days preceding, only now I would feel like I wasn't myself—almost like I was looking at my life from outside my own body. I would know who I was and where everything was in my house, but I wouldn't feel like it was *me*. At some point the dizziness would get so bad I couldn't even stand. Then my vision would start to go a little funky—almost like I was losing it. The center of my vision would actually disappear. It didn't turn black, it just wasn't there. I could only see things with my peripheral vision.

About an hour afterward, I would begin to feel nauseous. Sometimes I vomited. Then the head pounding would begin. All I could do was to take some Excedrin, lie down in a dark room, and wait for it to pass. My migraines would last a long and tiring eight hours, on average. Then I would have about a month's time before the next one would come.

—N.G.

The third phase of migraine is the *headache* itself, which can last anywhere from four hours to three days. Those with migraine-based head pain will often have pain on just one side (although up to 40 percent can experience pain on both sides). And this pain is significant—a 5 to 10 on a "10" pain scale. It is of a pulsing or throbbing quality, and it is increased by physical movement or exertion. That is why most people prefer to lie very still during a migraine attack. It is during this phase when *allodynia* (described earlier) can become a significant factor for some.

The final phase of migraine is known as the *postdrome*. After the floodwaters of head pain finally recede, a migraineur is often left in one of two extreme states. Either they feel completely drained by the ordeal; or they feel perfectly euphoric, proclaiming, "Thank God it's over!"

Migraine Without Aura

In the past, you may have had a well-meaning but ill-informed person tell you that the headaches you suffer couldn't be migraines, because you lack the pre-headache nausea and flashing-lights phenomena. This couldn't be further from the truth. Migraines without aura are actually very common, and they are indeed migraines. Here is an example of a fellow church member of mine who deals with them.

I do not remember when my headaches first began, but I do remember being most affected by them in the ninth grade. I missed quite a bit of school that year. When I had a headache, I couldn't bear to sit under the fluorescent lights or to be around the loud noises that were typical of a large high school. My mother took me to our family physician, a chiropractor, and ultimately to a neurologist. It was the neurologist who finally diagnosed my headaches as "neck-related migraines." (He discovered a "knot" in the top of my neck right under the back of my skull the size of a golf ball!) He started me on a migraine medication, amitriptyline, which I took at each mealtime and before bed. While I was on it, my migraines decreased in severity and frequency. However, when I attempted to go off the medication three months later, my migraines returned to their premedicated state.

I have continued to deal with periodic migraines for the last 18 years. Whenever I sense a migraine coming on, it usually begins with an aching in my upper neck (at the base of the skull on both sides of my spine). Soon afterward, I feel a tremendous pressure and tightening in the same area of my neck. I've come to expect that this pain and pressure will spread over the top and side of my head until it settles behind one of my eyes. During a migraine attack, bright lights, loud noises, and any movement will cause my head pain and pressure to increase dramatically—to the point where I almost cannot breathe. Nausea commonly occurs with my migraines, as does dizziness and a general feeling of weakness all over my body.

Throughout most of those years, I self-treated my head pain with ibuprofen, ice, and rest. This regime would help decrease the severity of my head pain, but would not always eliminate the migraine completely. In 2006, I began to realize that many of my migraines were related to my menstrual cycle—usually coming two to three days prior to its beginning. When I reported this to my gynecologist, he prescribed Imitrex, another migraine medication. I was told to use this medicine (an injection) at the first sign of a migraine. Imitrex is supposed to abort my headache altogether. Unfortunately, my most recent migraine had me in bed for three days and taking the Imitrex three times before it finally subsided!

While most of my migraines will respond to Imitrex, I do not like the side effects of this drug. At this time, I'm awaiting results of other health tests before I begin to seek further treatment. I'm realizing my migraines are occurring more regularly and with much greater severity, so I feel it's time for me to do some further investigating.

—A.S.

Migraine *Without* Headache

You heard me correctly—I said migraine *without* headache. While this is certainly unusual, I've treated two such patients over the years. The medical term is *ocular migraines*. In these cases, the brain goes through the sequence of events I described in the beginning of this chapter. When the electrical wave of heightened activity, followed by decreased activity, sweeps across the brain's surface, visual disturbances are experienced. But then the brain somehow aborts the process, and the person does not progress into the throbbing headache or the postdrome phases. Here is the story of one such patient.

The first time I experienced an ocular migraine, I was driving in the car. My clear vision suddenly became partially obstructed. After rubbing my eyes to clear what I thought was debris, I quickly realized it was my vision. This scared me, so I pulled the car to the side of the road.

The best way I can describe this vision problem is to say it was as if I were looking through a kaleidoscope filled with wiggling worms rather than brightly colored plastic pieces. If I tilted my head, the orientation of the "worms" would change. They were mostly in my peripheral vision. If I looked straight ahead, I could see clearly. This lasted about 20 minutes.

A month or so later the same thing happened again. This prompted me to visit my eye doctor and eventually a neurologist. My condition was diagnosed as ocular migraines—migraines with visual aura, but without the headache.

—P.J.

It is now recognized that P.J.'s visual symptoms were due to the increased electrical activity sweeping across his brain's surface. What is not understood is why this electrical activity leads to so many different visual experiences (starbursts, jagged lines, "worms," and such). Another patient of mine who suffered with ocular migraines would experience a total loss of vision that would last 20 to 30 minutes. This phenomenon was caused by the secondary decrease in brain's electrical activity.

When Cluster Headaches Gang Up on You

Back when I was in school, training to become a physical therapist, I clearly remember my professor describing cluster headaches. She told us they were nicknamed "suicide headaches" because the pain was so severe (10 on a pain scale of "10")—and the episodes so unrelenting—that people had been known to take their own lives rather than continue living with (and in fear of) them.

Cluster headaches are so named because they occur in a clustered or grouped fashion. The first headache episode, which lasts from 15 to 90 minutes, is followed by another episode within the next one to eight days, followed by a third, and so on. This headache pattern continues for a period of two weeks to three months, and then, as abruptly as it began, it goes away. The headaches may vanish for a year and then, out of the blue, they're back with a vengeance. And the cycle resumes.

The pain of a typical cluster headache is experienced on one side of the head, in either the temple or the eye area or sometimes both. The pain quality is described as a sharp stabbing or burning. Because of the extreme severity of pain, a cluster-headache sufferer will anxiously pace during an attack, unlike the migraineur, who will want to lie perfectly still. Associated with this pain is one or more of the following symptoms occurring on the same side of the head: eye tearing; eyelid swelling or drooping; nose congestion or running. The eye and nose conditions come about via the trigeminal nerve and its brain connection, the trigeminal-cervical nucleus (TCN—refer back to figure 3.7).

Science has been specifically targeting an area in the brain called the *hypothalamus* as the source of the cluster headache. The hypothalamus, among other things, controls our wake–sleep cycles. This area is under scrutiny because a cluster headache will often begin while a person is asleep.

Today, medication and other treatments are available that can ease and shorten the suffering experienced during an attack. (See chapter 11, "Prescription for Relief.") Unfortunately, no cures have been discovered, and there is still very little known about why these headaches occur. The following is an account of a cluster-headache experience.

> Cluster headaches began for me when I was 28 years old. The first time one occurred I thought I was getting a regular ol' headache. So I popped a bunch of aspirin and waited. Strangely, it was on just one side of my head, so I dismissed it as sinus pressure—hey, I was young and healthy, what else could it be?
>
> For two years I went without a headache—until one day it was back, and again, only on my right side. Remembering my self-diagnosis of sinus pressure from the last go-round, I began taking Actifed. Over the next two weeks I endured these headaches, which would come on and off throughout the day. By week three they stopped, so I never went to the doctor.
>
> Following three years of being head-pain-free, my headache returned with a vengeance! It was so sharp and so sudden that

I went immediately to my doctor. The best way I can describe it is that it felt as if someone had grabbed me from behind and begun stabbing me, in and around my right eye, with an ice pick—twisting it until I could almost feel it come out the back of my head (where my neck meets my skull). After 30 to 40 minutes of this torture, I would be released from my tormentor's grasp. My doctor placed me on antibiotics (in case of a sinus infection) and ordered an MRI, a CT scan, and an EEG. He also referred me to a neurologist. When all my tests and examinations came back negative, I was given a "clean bill of health." One month from the time this headache cycle began, it ended.

Two years later, you guessed it…my headache was back. I tried everything I could think of when the pain came. I put burning hot compresses against my eye, stuck my head in the freezer, and popped four and five Advils at a time. I paced the streets at night—since you can't possibly sit still when this kind of pain hits! My right eye would get blood-red and weep continuously. My right sinus felt as if was going to explode. One time, out of desperation, I began banging the back of my head against something, only to find later that I had cut my head open. The pain of the wound obviously didn't compare with my eye pain.

What made this headache cycle different from the previous ones was the availability of information on the Internet. I began searching for answers and discovered that what I was experiencing was known as cluster headaches. I learned of the drug Imitrex, which was being effectively used for treatment. I got a prescription as fast as I could. It was a godsend! It acted so fast, and I could continue on with my sleep or my day's activities. Unfortunately, this particular cluster cycle dragged on for much longer than my previous cycles. I was in my fifth month of clusters when I discovered (again through the Internet) the problem of rebound headaches sometimes caused by these medications. I went cold turkey, and after suffering through two more bouts, I was again headache-free.

Online, I was amazed to find that many others were suffering with this same horrible sentence. Through a chat room of fellow "clusterheads" I was able to contact another sufferer. As a result I found out about his treatment regime, which included verapamil and inhalation of pure oxygen. I went straight to my doctor and asked him to prescribe the same for me. This has been the most effective treatment to date for me. I know if I act immediately, I can stop the pain within five minutes! I am so thankful to finally be able to control this pain, instead of it controlling me.

Brain-Pain Triggers

The way in which Webster's dictionary describes *trigger* is "to initiate, activate, or set off; to cause the explosion of." If that second part of the definition isn't descriptive of a migraine or cluster headache, I don't know what is! A headache trigger is a preceding factor which *sets off* or *initiates* a headache "explosion." Typically it takes more than one trigger to be present for a headache to develop, but in some highly sensitive people it may take only one. Even though the triggers of migraine and cluster headaches may overlap somewhat, more is known (or, should I say, suspected) about migraine triggers.

Migraine Triggers

If you have done any reading about migraines in books or magazine articles, they always include a list of common migraine triggers. Here you will likely find such things as

- bright, flashing lights
- loud noise
- strong odors (perfume, gasoline, and so on)
- stress
- inadequate sleep
- hormone-level change (in females, estrogen-level drop prior to menses)
- certain foods—namely red wine, aged cheese, chocolate, caffeine, and anything containing MSG or nitrates—but the list goes on further

Many of the above triggers are agreed upon by scientists and physicians alike. But controversy does exist as to whether or not the above named foods are truly *triggers*—or simply *cravings* associated with the prodrome phase (which takes place between one to three days prior to the headache phase). Let me explain. If you eat a chocolate bar a day before your migraine, you may think the chocolate is a trigger. You may even have found it to be a recurring situation. Every time you indulge in a chocolate bar, you wind up with a headache the next day.

Alternatively, what if your brain feels a drop in its levels of serotonin (a chemical that's suspected to be related to the initiation of brain pain in migraines and cluster headaches). In response your brain sends you a message: "You must find and eat some chocolate" (since chocolate consumption has been proved to increase the body's serotonin level). Maybe instead of being a trigger, your chocolate craving and subsequent consumption was your brain's way of trying to defuse an oncoming headache. (The only way to know with any level of certainty is to perform an experiment on yourself. You'll find it described in chapter 9.)

There are a couple of migraine-triggers that may come as a surprise to you, and even to your doctor. First, studies have shown that migraineurs have more migraines during times of *wet weather* patterns. Unfortunately, barring a move to a desert climate like that of Las Vegas or Phoenix, you don't have much recourse here.

Second, the trigger least commonly associated with migraines—and the one you have most potential to do something about—is *upper-neck joint, disc, and muscle dysfunction.* (See chapters 3 through 6, where I related this to neck-based headaches.) Amazingly, I have achieved extraordinary clinical success in ending migraine headaches by helping my brain-pain patients with these same tools and techniques! In the next chapter you'll find three remarkable, hope-breeding migraineur success stories related to this upper neck trigger. So do yourself a big favor. If you suffer from migraines, get to a physical practitioner who is trained to resolve problems in the upper neck. It may be the key to unlocking your migraines, as so many of my patients have found.

Are Migraines Truly "All in Your Head"?

In 2006, an important study demonstrated a high correlation of neck "issues" in the unilateral (one-sided) migraine population when they were compared with healthy subjects. This finding was reported in the medical journal *Cephalgia* ("head pain") by César Fernández-de-las-Peñas, PT. His research confirmed that migraine patients had a *greater number of active trigger points in the muscles on the same side as their migraines.* Also noted was that migraine sufferers had 1) a greater degree of forward posture and 2) decreased neck mobility when compared with nonmigraineurs.

Still left unanswered is the question: Does a migraine create these neck findings, or do problems in the neck set off a migraine? Though this is a necessary query for future research, clinically I've seen migraines resolved by eliminating their associated trigger points and improving head posture and neck mobility—and that is enough for me and my patients!

Cluster-Headache Triggers

Although not much is known about cause and effect within the cluster-headache population, some correlations have surfaced with enough regularity to be called triggers. They include

- alcohol consumption
- smoking tobacco
- stress
- sleep deprivation
- possibly, seasonal sensitivities (for instance, in autumn or spring)

The good news is, all of these triggers can be avoided or managed, unlike many of the migraineurs' triggers.

Headache Thresholds—When the Triggers Add Up

The *threshold* is the point at which your headache begins. As we've already established, those of you with brain pain have lower headache thresholds than those who do not. Then there are those few superhumans who never get headaches. (Boy, I wish I were one of them!) They would be said to have extremely high headache thresholds, so high that they never seem to reach the doorway to headache land at all.

The illustration below shows you how individual headache triggers can add up, and how experiencing the "required" number of triggers simultaneously will produce a headache. You will note that not only is a brain-pain headache sufferer's "stick of dynamite" bigger (hence yielding a more powerful headache explosion), but their "fuse" is also much shorter (indicating a lowered headache threshold).

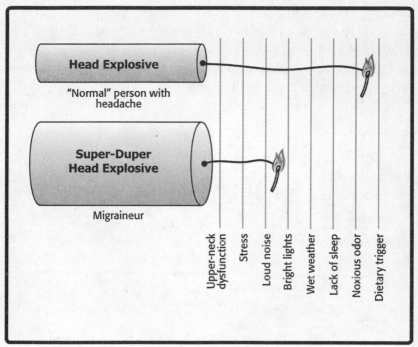

figure 8.1

Certain medications—discussed in chapter 11—can act to lengthen your "fuse" and therefore increase the number of triggers you can tolerate before head pain ensues. If we think about this relationship between trigger build up and headache threshold (tolerance*) in terms of percentages, we could draw this analogy:

---

* *Tolerance* refers to *adaptability*—the ability to absorb insults (stresses) without experiencing injury (pain).

Brain-pain patient without preventative meds = 50% tolerance to triggers
Brain-pain patient taking preventative meds   = 65% tolerance to triggers
"Normal" headache response   = 80% tolerance to triggers
"Superhuman, brain like steel"   = 100% tolerance to triggers

A holistic approach to your brain-pain treatment will likely need to be twofold. First, you must determine and decrease your known triggers. Secondly, you will need to try to increase your headache threshold. While only medication is known to desensitize your brain (increase your threshold), you can play a significant role in eliminating or decreasing your headache frequency by knowing what "gets on your brain's nerves" and working to eliminate those things. Follow me through the next three chapters. There's much that can be done to affect your brain pain in positive ways.

Chapter 9

Figuring Out Your Triggers

With so many triggers mentioned in the last chapter, how in the world will you be able to uncover what your personal triggers are? Not a problem. In this chapter, after we discuss each of the most common triggers in more detail, you'll find out how to investigate each one to see if it has a negative impact on your headaches. Next, I'll offer practical suggestions on how to avoid those triggers, when possible, as well as give you ways to deal with the triggers you are unable to modify on your own.

In treating migraines, there are significant trigger modifications and elimination techniques available to you. It is my belief that the *first* course of action in migraine treatment should not include medication. Medicine should be reserved for when nothing else is working or when other self-management options have left you with partial but unsatisfactory results. It's better to approach brain pain with less invasive methods before moving into the realm of medications (prescription or over-the-counter).

Because I know that many people will still need to supplement trigger modification with medication, chapter 11 will provide you with a thorough survey of the medications in use today for migraine and cluster headache management, including both their pros (targeted purposes) and cons (side effects). But for now, let's see what can be done to defuse your brain pain before taking a trip to the drugstore or pharmacy.

Long-term Issues

Medications, while often effective, are somewhat toxic to the body. Some have an effect on the liver, others on the kidneys. Many will affect your brain's chemistry (serotonin levels). Long-term use can possibly create other health concerns down the road. I say this to make you aware, not to scare you away from using such medicines. All medications in use today in the United States are FDA-approved. And if I could not get relief from migraine or cluster headache pain any other way, you can bet I'd be at the pharmacy in a flash!

Keeping Track of Your Headaches

In order to determine what your particular head-pain triggers are, you'll need to become an investigative reporter of sorts. You must diligently record all the details surrounding each of your headaches. While you think you could never forget your last headache, you will, in part. Whenever I take a verbal history during my patients' evaluation, I am many times surprised at how little they recall about their own pain. People often have difficulty telling me when their last pain episode began, when or what made it worse, where it began, and how long it lasted. All they know for sure is that they have pain and that it's interfering with their lives.

The first thing I ask each patient to do is to keep a record of their headaches for me. I have provided an easy-to-use headache tracker chart for you below. Keep it with you during the day and at your bedside at night, and diligently fill it out. If you've not yet seen a neurologist or physical practitioner, having this with you will prove beneficial. Your health-care provider will know you mean business and that you will be carefully monitoring your treatment outcome. It will also provide clues and evidence as to what intervention is working for you and what is not. I suggest you keep a log of your headaches until they are a thing of the past (or at least down to the point where you can enjoy most of your life again).

Migraine and Cluster-Headache Tracker

Month: _____

Day of the month	Intensity (1-10)	Duration (number of hours)	Pain location and quality	Environmental factors (lights, sounds, and so on)	Associated symptoms (see list below)
1					
2					
3					
4					
5					
6					
7					
8					
9					
10					
11					
12					
13					
14					
15					
16					

A. stiff or painful neck
B. nausea
C. vomiting
D. visual disturbances*
E. sensitivity to bright lights
F. sensitivity to loud noises

G. nasal stuffiness
H. runny nose
I. sensitivity to strong odors
J. tingling (pins and needles)
K. eye tearing
L. eyelid swelling

M. face drooping
N. numbness (loss of sensation)
O. fatigue, yawning
P. agitation
Q. loss of part of your visual field

* Visual disturbances include flashing, blinking lights, and distorted images.

Migraine and Cluster-Headache Tracker

Month: _____

Day of the month	Intensity (1-10)	Duration (number of hours)	Pain location and quality	Environmental factors (lights, sounds, and so on)	Associated symptoms (see list below)
17					
18					
19					
20					
21					
22					
23					
24					
25					
26					
27					
28					
29					
30					
31					

A. stiff or painful neck
B. nausea
C. vomiting
D. visual disturbances*
E. sensitivity to bright lights
F. sensitivity to loud noises

G. nasal stuffiness
H. runny nose
I. sensitivity to strong odors
J. tingling (pins and needles)
K. eye tearing
L. eyelid swelling

M. face drooping
N. numbness (loss of sensation)
O. fatigue, yawning
P. agitation
Q. loss of part of your visual field

* Visual disturbances include flashing, blinking lights, and distorted images.

Exposing Possible Migraine Triggers:
Making the Con-NECK-tion

For nearly 20 years now I have been treating patients with headaches, most of which stemmed from either an acute neck injury (such as whiplash) or a chronic neck-pain situation. The majority of them were referred to me by their doctors. For this reason, their headaches were typically cervicogenic in origin.

Recently, however, I have been offering my manual PT services to people who suffer from migraine headaches. In doing so, I have made a wonderful discovery. By treating the upper-neck joint, muscle, and disc dysfunctions of this group, I have been able to eliminate *all* of their migraines! Yes—these people's migraines do not merely decrease in frequency or intensity, they are *eliminated*. (Do I hear a hallelujah? I know I did from those patients!)

Credit Where Credit Is Due

Back in the early 1990s I worked at a facility that hosted a headache center. In this center, a physical therapist (occasionally me) and a neurologist would co-evaluate patients suffering from different forms of headache. The PT would assess the patient's posture and muscle quality in the head, face, and neck areas, and perform a detailed jaw (if warranted) and spinal examination of the neck and upper back. The neurologist would perform his neurological assessment and order any tests he deemed necessary. After consultation between the PT and the neurologist, joint recommendations were made for physical therapy, stress management, medication, and so on—whatever was considered best for that particular patient.

As a result of the mentoring I received from the center's co-director, Howard Makofsky, DHSc, PT, OCS, I started on the road to successful treatment within the headache population. I owe my knowledge of neck-based headache causes and manual treatments primarily to him.

I have three stories of hope I'd like to share with you. Each migraine sufferer has found relief in the hands of a physical practitioner who addressed their upper-neck issues. I know after reading these stories you'll understand and begin to believe in the *con-NECK-tion* as well.

From a Migraineur Without Aura

Over the past year or two, my headaches had begun occurring with such frequency (three to four times a week and sometimes daily) that the amount of medication I was taking was beginning to scare me. I knew I had to do something else to get to the bottom of why I was really getting these headaches.

I had done everything I knew to do. Originally, I had seen my general practitioner. He directed me to a neurologist who specialized in migraine headaches. The neurologist ordered an MRI and other brain scans just to rule out other more significant problems. All the tests came back negative.

One day, while discussing my predicament with several friends, they encouraged me to try chiropractic treatment (all of these friends were being treated by the same chiropractor for different reasons). They seemed certain their chiropractor could help my situation. I had always been skeptical about chiropractic treatment, although I don't really know why. When I dragged my feet in following through with my friends' advice, it was my husband who took the initiative to call and make an appointment for my evaluation.

I have to say that even after the chiropractor declared that there was a very clear reason why I was getting headaches (my spine was in bad shape) and that it was definitely treatable, I remained skeptical. I knew that the proof was only going to come by giving myself completely over to the treatment plan she recommended for me. My treatment recommendation was to come in for an "adjustment" [*] of my neck three times a week in addition to doing some home exercises. Secondly, she asked me to stop taking my medications. She said that I basically needed to clean out my body of all the drugs I had taken. As we went along in the adjustments, if I did get a migraine, I could come in and see her every day, if need be, until the headache was gone.

I began my treatment plan on September 18, 2006. After eight months of treatment, astoundingly I have had only three

---

* See upper cervical spine manipulation precautions in chapter 7.

major headaches and only a smattering of minor headaches! I must admit the first three months of treatment were a little tough without all my medications and such, but I was able to get through this time with the help of my chiropractor. I am thrilled that my treatment was finally able to get to the root of the migraines instead of just treating the symptoms with narcotic medications.

—F.M.

This story was provided by a friend of mine who chose to go the chiropractic route after having tried physical therapy to no avail. Not all physical practitioners are created equal—this woman saw a physical therapist who did not know how to treat the dysfunctions in her upper neck. I'm glad she found someone who could help her. Although, after eight months of treatment she is still experiencing some migraines, on the upside, she has been freed from most medication, and her overall headache frequency and intensity are much improved.

From a Migraineur with Aura

I think my mom got tired of watching me crack my neck. She asked her friend (the author of this book) if there was anything she could do to help me with my neck problem. Lisa agreed to take a look at me. During my physical therapy evaluation, she became aware that not only was I having daily neck pain, but I was also experiencing monthly premenstrual migraines.

Lisa taught me a lot about my headaches, like how my neck pain could possibly trigger a migraine. After working on my neck, she taught me some exercises that I should do at home whenever I would feel the urge to crack my neck. Typically I would feel like my neck was getting tighter toward the late afternoon. So when that time came, I did her stretches. And my neck gradually began to feel better. After a week or so, I noticed that I didn't need to stretch as often as I did at first.

My migraines, although not instantly gone, did get shorter and shorter. They went from lasting eight hours to only about three. This was a big relief for me. After a month or so of treatment, my migraines went away completely! At first, I would wait anxiously each month for my premenstrual headache to begin. But to my surprise it never happened. I've gone over a year now without getting so much as one migraine!

—N.G.

This story was written by a former patient of mine. As for her physical therapy regime, I saw her for a total of nine treatments, once a week. After the ninth visit, she was discharged with a home program to maintain her status. I do get to ask her from time to time about her migraines. Happily, she continues to report their nonexistence—two years later! This is life-changing news! All I can do is write about it and hope the person who needs the information will get it. Please, if you know someone else who is suffering with migraines, offer them what you've learned here. Give them this book as a gift! They will be forever in your debt if this is the key that unlocks them from their years of pain.

From a Migraineur Without Headache

One evening at a church function, I was standing around chatting with my friend Lisa (the author of this book). She was telling me about her latest writing project. My eyes lit up. "I've been getting these awful vision problems. It's pretty scary when it happens, especially if I happen to be driving. My doc says they're ocular migraines and there's really nothing I can do about them." Lisa smiled and said, "Let's not draw that conclusion so quickly. Why don't you come into my office and I'll treat your neck, and we'll see what happens. Maybe I could help you." Well, I quickly followed her advice.

During my first visit, Lisa found I had some joint and muscle problems in my upper neck that she said she could fix. I also told her that, in addition to the weird eye-symptom episodes, I had also awakened with severe headaches on average three to four times per month for as long as I could remember.

Lisa finished her evaluation and got to work on my neck that same day. She gave me some posture suggestions and some neck stretches to do at home. When I returned for my next visit, a week later, I reported that I had remained headache- and eye-symptom-free since the day of my evaluation. Lisa treated me a total of five or six times. I've never had another headache or ocular migraine episode since!

—P.J.

Pretty amazing stories, aren't they? I am utterly convinced that all migraineurs should seek evaluation and treatment of their necks.* It could quite possibly be all you need to do. Wouldn't that be simply wonderful?

---

* Again, see chapter 7, "Putting Yourself in the Hands of a Professional," for guidance.

Chapter 10

Defusing Your Triggers

After finishing this chapter and the previous one, I hope you'll be seeing the full picture of ways you can defuse your headache triggers without medication. The fact is, there are many nonmedicinal options for overcoming migraines and even cluster headaches. Investigating them will require time and effort, but the rewards are too great for you to not pursue each possibility.

You already know that I feel it's critical to start defusing your triggers by seeking neck evaluation. This chapter continues with other triggers that you will need to consider identifying and controlling.

Protecting Your Senses

...From Noise

Who besides teenagers thrills to loud, continuous auditory assaults? What is pleasurable "head-banging" music for a teen creates a different sort of head-banging for a migraineur. There is universal agreement that loud, unremitting noise can bring on a migraine. So whether we're talking about music, noise in confined spaces such as a car or an airplane, or outdoor noise like that found at a sporting event, or simply walking down a city sidewalk ears ringing with the sound of traffic horns and jackhammers, all these ear assaults can set off your brain pain in no time flat.

If this is one of your triggers, you know that full well. While your best bet is to avoid loud noises, this is in many instances quite

151

impossible. What I am suggesting is that you think ahead and prepare yourself for the assault. You need ear armor. This ear gear comes in many forms. You can get yourself some earplugs, wear earmuffs in the winter, or buy a pair of those fancy noise-canceling headphones (great for airplanes, long car rides, and so on). When you can't avoid the noise, you must somehow shield yourself from its force.

...From Visual Sources

Bright or strobing (pulsing) lights are another known trigger for migraines. When bright light is the problem, sunglasses are the answer. Better still, get a pair of polarized sunglasses. These really cut down on glare, as they block out 50 percent of the light rays that beam toward your eyes. In addition to the polarized lenses, these glasses also have a shaded tint, which dims the remaining light rays. If you work under fluorescent lights, which also have a strobing effect, see if you can switch them off and use incandescent lighting instead.

For those of you who work staring at a computer screen as part of your job (my buddies), I've been told by my software-engineer husband that your computer monitor can be adjusted in such a way as to decrease its ability to trigger your oversensitive brain. Bear with me now as I give a simplified, secondhand explanation of what the problem with computer screens is and what you can do about it.

Traditional, non-flat-screen computer monitors emit light by way of a cathode-ray tube, or CRT. The CRT's job is to "redraw" the images that are on your screen at scheduled time intervals. As the rays rapidly sweep across the screen, "refreshing" your material, your eyes pick up this refreshing as a flicker of light. At lower refresh rate settings (greater time in between "refreshings"), the flickering can trigger a migraine for some. The higher the refresh rate, the harder it is to perceive the flicker; therefore, the better it is for your eyes (and brain).

A typical curved-screen monitor may have a refresh rate of 65Hz. Maximum tops out at 80 to 85Hz. The rate is typically adjustable and depends on both the computer and the monitor capabilities. Instructions on setting the refresh rate will be different depending upon your computer make and model and the software running on it. (Refer to your "help" files or your local techie for assistance here.) I have also been told—again by my hubby—that a flat-screen monitor is a much better choice for a migraineur because it does not have the same refreshing issues as a CRT screen.

...From Scents

Finally, another possible migraine trigger that attacks your senses is...scent. Strong odors, whether intended for good (perfumes or air fresheners) or regularly encountered as the by-product of the environment in which you live (gasoline, secondhand smoke, or car exhaust fumes) can all send brain-pain-stimulating messages right through your nose!

How do you combat these? The first thing you can do is make family, friends, and coworkers aware of your migraine trigger and ask (nicely) if they might consider refraining from wearing strong scents or smoking where you can smell the fumes. If you are triggered by gasoline (I am right there with you), use full-serve-only gas pumps and keep your windows closed. Other outdoor smells can be less offensive when breathed in through a scarf-barrier. (However, if it's not the wintertime, this suggestion can look a bit odd.)

Other Triggering Circumstances

Guard Your Sleep

Oh, the trouble a bad night's sleep can cause! A tired brain is a more irritable brain—just like a tired momma is easily set off by her kids. We cannot always fight against insomnia, which visits most people at some time or another. Yet there are a number of things you can do to stack the odds of getting a restful sleep in your favor:

- Maintain a regular lights-off bedtime. (This time should be seven to eight hours earlier than your alarm clock rings the next morning.)
- Do something restful, like reading, before you turn off the lights. Television-watching, while you may believe it helps you unwind, often stimulates your brain.

- Do not drink or eat caffeinated items after 6 p.m.
- Do not have emotional encounters before going to bed. (This is not the time to discuss finances with your spouse.)
- Don't drink excessively in the evening. This will help you to avoid the bladder wake-up call at 3 a.m.
- Avoid spicy foods after dinnertime. No one sleeps well with an agitated stomach lining.

Bad Weather

Studies have demonstrated that wet-weather patterns can stir up a migraine. Here's the thing. We live on planet Earth. We are bound to experience bad weather. One could up and move to the desert, but let's be real. This is a nice trigger-fact, but that's all. My hope is that when you decrease some of your other adjustable triggers, the only influence wet weather will have on you is to send you looking for your umbrella.

Emotional Upset

Emotions play a huge role in our physical health. So it isn't surprising that negative emotions such as anger and anxiety can trigger a migraine. I do not have a quick Band-Aid suggestion for dealing with these two strong emotions (nor does anyone else!). For this reason, I've devoted the last chapter of this book, "Navigating Through the Seas of Discontent," to an in-depth discussion of these powerful feelings and their effect on head pain.

Food: Good for the Stomach, Bad for the Brain?

Every source I've studied in preparation for writing this book includes a superlong list of foods recognized to be triggers for *some* migraine sufferers. Invariably, the list ends with a statement like "...and any other foods you've found that trigger your headaches." While I will provide you with a similar list, keep in mind that even the most common brain-pain-triggering substances may not have any effect on you.

The importance in familiarizing yourself with what is on the dietary triggers list is twofold. First, you can know which edible substances to be wary of, and second, you can know what foods to cut out of your diet if you seek to follow the "Migraine Diet" method I'll describe later in this chapter. (By the way, most lists tell you what to avoid. For optimism's sake, I've included a list, alongside, of better options.)

Dietary Considerations

Dietary Triggers[8]	Possible "Fuse Igniters"	Better Options
Aged cheeses	Parmesan, Romano, sour cream, cheddar, and the like	Fresh mozzarella, ricotta, cream cheese, provolone
Alcohol	Red wine, champagne, dark liquors	White wine, vodka
Beans	Fava, lima, navy, pinto, pod, string, lentils	Red kidney, black, garbanzo (chickpeas)
Caffeine	Coffee, tea (iced and hot), hot chocolate, energy drinks	Decaffeinated versions
Chocolate	Solid, liquid, or icing form	White "chocolate"
Fruits and their juices	Citrus (oranges, pineapples, grapefruits, lemons, limes), dried fruits, avocados, bananas, figs, dates, papaya, red raspberries, red plums	Apples, mangos, melons, strawberries, blueberries, green grapes, peaches
MSG	Chinese food, canned soups, croutons or canned bread crumbs, ready-prepared foods (check labels)	Fresh, homemade alternatives
Nitrates	Pepperoni, salami, bologna, bacon, hot dogs	Fresh-sliced chicken, turkey, ham, or roast beef
Nuts	Peanut butter and nut mixes	Seeds (sunflower, pumpkin)
Onions	White, yellow, and red	Chives, leeks, scallions, shallots
Processed meats and fish	Beef jerky, dried sausage, lox, pickled herring, anchovies	Fresh fish, canned tuna or salmon
Sweeteners	Nutrasweet, Sweet 'n' Low	Stevia, Splenda
Yeast-raised baked goods	Freshly baked bread, doughnuts, pizza dough, pretzels that are less than a day old	Anything more than one day old
Vinegar	Balsamic, red wine	White wine, apple-cider

Addressing Your Food Triggers: Keeping a Food Journal

An effective way to identify your "edible irritants" is to keep a food journal. I have designed one, which can be found on the next few pages. You'll need to diligently record all you eat and drink and compare it with your headache-tracker chart (pages 143–144). Only then will you uncover any correlation between what goes in your mouth and what goes on between your ears.

Food Journal

Month: _____

Day of the month	Breakfast	Lunch	Dinner	Snacks
1				
2				
3				
4				
5				
6				
7				
8				
9				
10				

Food Journal

Month: _____

Day of the month	Breakfast	Lunch	Dinner	Snacks
11				
12				
13				
14				
15				
16				
17				
18				
19				
20				
21				

Food Journal

Month: _____

Day of the month	Breakfast	Lunch	Dinner	Snacks
22				
23				
24				
25				
26				
27				
28				
29				
30				
31				

Addressing Your Food Triggers: The Migraine Diet

The confusing part of addressing your food triggers comes when you understand that, based on the threshold model, a food or drink that resulted in a headache last week may not have the same result this week because of the absence of other triggers. (Remember that triggers add up until they reach your unique "fuse-ignition level.") For this reason, some headache specialists have decided the best way to deal with food triggers needs to be total elimination...for a time.

This is the chosen method of neurologist Dr. David Buchholz. In his book *Heal Your Headache: The 1-2-3 Program for Taking Charge of Your Pain,* the method of the "Migraine Diet" is proposed. It really makes a great deal of sense. Because food triggers can be so very difficult to nail down, you must employ a drastic approach if any insight is to be gained. Dr. Buchholz asks his headache patients to abstain from *all* known food triggers, *all at once.* If headache improvement is noted after two months of abstinence from the suspected dietary triggers, the patient is encouraged to continue on the Migraine Diet for two more months, bringing the total abstaining period to four months.

At that point, the patient is told to add back their most favorite (and sorely missed) item from the list. They are instructed to eat it every day for one week. If no headaches have occurred, then another previously avoided food can be reintroduced to the migraineur's menu. If, however, a headache does develop, that dietary item remains "forbidden," and another food is given a try for a week. One by one, foods can be reintroduced, all the while maintaining a good scientific handle on what items are one's personal triggers and should therefore be avoided.[9] This is indeed a long process, but Dr. Buchholz claims the results are worth the diligence.

I am not so naïve as to think every migraineur can find complete relief without supplementing their care with medication or some other form of herbal or alternative treatment. For this reason, in the next chapter, I will specifically describe the current medications and alternative therapies available for the treatment of migraines.

Cluster-headache Triggers

Cluster-headache sufferers have a far simpler list of known influences when it comes to triggering headaches. (Unfortunately, the causes and processes of cluster headaches are still shrouded in mystery for the most part.) Their list of triggers includes

- aged meats
- alcohol
- bright lights
- cigarette and other tobacco smoke
- extremes of heat or cold
- "letdown" following high stress
- MSG (monosodium glutamate)

This list contains more easily avoidable irritants than does the heftier migraine-trigger list. According to *Migraine and Other Headaches* by Drs. William Young and Stephen Silberstein, cluster-headache sufferers are "often smokers and are (or have been) heavy drinkers."[10]

Scientific research is slim on cluster headaches likely because it is a rare head-pain condition, affecting only 1 in 1000 people. (Funding for studies typically follows the larger patient populations.) That does not mean these headaches are without known treatment. In the following chapter, I will devote a section to what medications are used when trying to combat and ease the pain of the cluster-headache cycle. This will be good news to those of you who suffer with this affliction.

Chapter 11

Prescription for Relief

Because medication types can be so confusing and their intended results are often poorly understood by the very patients who use them, this book would be incomplete if it did not include this chapter. Now, it is important to inform you, right from the get-go, that as a physical therapist, I am not licensed to prescribe or dispense either over-the-counter (OTC) or prescription medication. But it is my desire to provide brain-pain sufferers with a clear education on medication. So we will discuss which medications are typically prescribed for what condition, what the hoped-for results should be, and what not-so-welcomed side effects or contraindications exist, if any.

When you understand the ins and outs of the medicines you are taking, you can play a more vital role in working with your doctor to find the best drug and the best dosage to treat your headaches. So let's get started, shall we?

Finding the Right Physician

Your primary doctor's job is to screen your present head-pain complaint, treat what they feel needs only their attention and expertise, and decide whether or not to send you on for further lab testing or to be seen by a specialist.

If you are a patient who suffers with migraines or cluster-type headaches, your primary-care physician will likely refer you to a neurologist, a physician who specializes in the nervous system. The body's nervous system is comprised of the brain, the spinal cord, and all the nerves that travel out from these two structures having their affect in the farthest reaches of the body. Diseases that affect the nervous system are numerous (multiple sclerosis, Lou Gehrig's disease, or ALS, cerebral palsy, migraines, and so on).

Because there is such a vast array of ailments, neurologists sometimes specialize in one or two specific areas of diagnosis and treatment. This is not to say you *need* a neurologist who specializes specifically in headache, but it's best to not go straight to the first neurologist you find in the phone book. Personal recommendations are a good place to begin. Talk to other migraineurs you know. Ask them which neurologist manages their condition and if they are happy with the results. When people are happy with their doctors, praises gush from their mouths. If they simply shrug their shoulders and give you a flat response, keep searching.

If you are presently under the care of a neurologist and are not getting the results you seek, it is never too late to look further. One thing I know is, when a physician specializes in a concentrated area, such as headache management, they live, breathe, and eat headache treatment. By treating headache patients primarily, they get to see a broader range of headache variations and "difficult cases." This serves to improve their ability to prescribe effective head-pain treatment, especially when relief, in the past, has been elusive.

Finding a neurologist who specializes in headaches can sometimes be difficult. I suggest searching the Internet for local headache centers (which are typically hospital-based) or contacting one of the headache groups I've listed in the back of this book to see if they might be able to recommend a neurologist in your area.

Migraine Management

Over-the-Counter Medicines

Without exception, the migraineurs I have spoken with report their first course of action against their headaches came in the form of over-the-counter (OTC) medication. Each day on television, on the Internet, or in magazines, you will find advertisements for OTC drugs that purport to be *the* "headache-stopper." Some products have even added the "migraine" tag to their claims of relief. Depending on the particular medication, you'll need to take two, four, six, or possibly even eight pills a day! Whatever the dosage, "real relief," they claim, is just a drugstore away. Notice they use the term *relief,* not *cure.* The ugly, unadvertised fact is that many of these OTC medicines *feed* the headache cycle (as discussed in chapter 2, "Drug-Rebound Headaches"), making them more a part of the problem rather than the solution.

The two main types of OTC pain medicines available for headaches are *analgesics* (pain relievers) and *nonsteroidal anti-inflammatory drugs* (NSAIDS—medications that reduce inflammation). The chart below has name-brand products presently on the market without a prescription.

Product Name	Analgesic	NSAIDS
Advil (ibuprofen)		X
Aleve (naproxen sodium)		X
Anacin (aspirin/caffeine)	X	
Bayer (aspirin)	X	
Excedrin (acetaminophen/aspirin/caffeine)	X	
Ibuprofen		X
Motrin (ibuprofen)		X
Tylenol (acetaminophen)	X	

The upside of OTC medicines is that they are available without a prescription and are relatively inexpensive. However, even drugs that are approved by the government and made available for self-prescription can have harmful side effects. Studies have shown that prolonged or excessive use of Tylenol (acetaminophen) can lead to liver inflammation and eventually to cirrhosis (a scarring condition of the liver that renders it ineffective, eventually leading to death)—especially if you happen to drink alcohol as well. Chronic acetaminophen dosing has also been shown to damage the kidneys.

Overuse of aspirin-based products and NSAIDS can wreak havoc on the lining of your stomach, leading to abdominal bleeding or stomach ulcers. (Many of my patients report not being able to "stomach" anti-inflammatory medications.) There are contraindications regarding heart disease and NSAIDS usage as well.

Further, OTC medicines can also "clash" with other medications you may be taking. Your best bet is to talk to your doctor or pharmacist about which medications (OTC and prescription combinations) are best for you in light of coexisting health issues.

Prescription Medication: Preventative

In the last three chapters we spoke about how to identify and decrease your headache triggers, thus lowering your susceptibility to getting headaches. Here's the equation again:

Triggers + lowered threshold = Brain-pain headache

Preventative medications are prescribed to be taken on a daily basis. This is the proactive approach. The primary purpose of taking these medications is to *raise your brain-pain-headache threshold.* They accomplish this by chemically attaching their tiny molecules to some of your brain's oversensitive pain-initiating receptor sites. This, in effect, makes your brain less reactive in the face of aggravating triggers.

This is great news for migraineurs and cluster-headache patients! And not only do preventative drugs act to *decrease the frequency* of headaches, they also *decrease the intensity* of head pain when it does occur. They aid in the effectiveness of other medications taken at the time of an attack because a weakened headache is easier to overcome with medication than a full-blown one. Many people don't like to have to take a medication every day of their lives, but given these significant benefits, who wouldn't sign on to this plan?

Interestingly, none of the medications in this preventative group were developed initially for use with headaches. They were what's known as "off-label" medications, meaning they were created and approved by the FDA for uses other than headache management. In recent years some off-label medications (such as Depakote and Topamax) have been approved by the FDA for headache treatment also. This does not suggest that the others are, in any way, unsafe for use with migraines or cluster headaches, but simply that they were not initially intended for this use.

So how in the world did they become some of the first go-to drugs for physicians treating brain pain? Well, their effectiveness was stumbled upon, quite by surprise, when patients who had been taking them for other reasons began reporting significant improvement in their headaches. Voilà! One by one, new headache-treatment options were born.

Antidepressants are the first such "off-label" medication category we'll look at. Please don't be taken aback if your physician suggests you begin taking them. He or she is not suggesting you are depressed and therefore have headaches. Rather, because these medications are formulated to change the brain's sensitivity to chemical bonding, they may be effective in blocking some of the preceding steps (chemical brain processes) that result in a headache for you. Promising results have been experienced by both migraine and cluster-type headache patients.

Anti-seizure medications, initially used for seizure disorders, reduce the brain's excitability (convulsive) factor. Through processes similar to the antidepressive medications, this group of medicines can desensitize your brain, which may increase your headache threshold. These medications are used to treat both migraine and cluster headaches.

Beta blockers, originally used for high blood pressure, are another group of off-label medicines that have shown promise when prescribed for migraine patients. Like the other preventative medicines available, beta blockers can be a helpful treatment option for many by raising their headache thresholds and decreasing the size of their sticks of "dynamite."

Calcium-channel blockers have shown effectiveness in the treatment of both migraine and cluster-headache patients alike. Once used only for management of high blood pressure, they are used successfully to elevate headache thresholds of migraineurs and cluster headache sufferers.

Nonsteroidal anti-inflammatory drugs (NSAIDS) have shown themselves most effective with two types of migraines: menstrual and exertion-related (post-exercise, sexual intercourse, and the like). By taking NSAIDS prior to the onset of one's menses or exertion activity, many people are able to prevent or decrease the intensity of a headache. (See OTC medication chart above for medication listings.) In addition to OTC NSAIDS, there are more powerful prescription varieties available. That said, most experts agree that NSAIDS—OTC or prescription-based—are not particularly helpful for other migraine or cluster-headache incidents.

The chart below lists, as of 2007, the available and most typically prescribed medications in the preventative category for migraine treatment.

Preventative Prescription Medications for Migraines

Medication Category	The Brand Name	Generic Form	The Good (bonuses)	The Bad (side effects)	The Ugly (precautions)
Antidepressants	Aventyl Elavil Pamelor Vivactil	nortriptyline amitriptyline nortriptyline protriptyline	Helpful with co-existing anxiety, depression, or insomnia	Constipation Dry mouth Sedation Weight gain	Co-existing glaucoma, high blood pressure, and urinary retention problems
Antiseizure	Depakote Topamax	divalproex topiramate	Useful with seizure disorders and manic-depressive illness	Fatigue Hair loss Kidney stones Nausea Tremor Weight gain	May lessen the effectiveness of oral contraceptives Pregnancy
Beta blockers	Corgard Inderal Timolide	nadolol propanolol timolol	Treats high blood pressure	Depression Fatigue Insomnia	Diabetes Depression Asthma Heart disease Older than 65
Calcium-channel blockers	Calan Isoptin Verelan	All are forms of verapamil	Treats high blood pressure	Constipation Leg swelling	Taking other heart medications

Prescription Medication: *Abortive*

Prevention aside, when it is clear that a migraine "funnel cloud" is fast approaching, what's a head-pain sufferer to do? Prior to 1973, the only option was to swallow some general-acting painkiller, either OTC pills (discussed above) or physician-prescribed narcotics (discussed below).

With the introduction of Cafergot in 1973 (a caffeine and ergotamine "cocktail"), the twisting funnel cloud seemed to have met its match. Together the caffeine and ergotamine functioned to shrink the swelling of the brain's inflamed blood vessels. The result was decreased head pain—and better still, decreased headache duration for many. Ergotamines begin working within a 30-to-60-minute window and continue to remain effective for three to four hours. Unfortunately, using this drug often brings the unwelcome side effects of nausea, vomiting, or both. So it often needs to be taken along with an antinausea medicine (see section below on anti-emetic medications).

In 1993, a new, chemically different, abortive wonder drug was introduced to the pharmaceutical market. Imitrex was to be self-injected into the thigh muscle as soon as a person was aware of an impending migraine. The clinical results were excellent. Over the next ten years, other *triptan* medications have made their way onto market (see the chart below). A whopping 80 percent of migraine sufferers find relief from medications in the triptan family! Because of the high success of triptan meds and their lower number of side effects and limitations when compared to ergotamines, triptans have become the abortive drug of choice since their introduction.

True Joy over Medication

Believe me when I say that for the first time ever, a new rainbow was on the horizon for migraineurs with the triptan medications. The first brand on the market was *Imitrex*. I remember its advent well. It occurred "back in the day," when I was seeing patients in my hospital's headache center. The center's neurologist, who was co-evaluating patients with me that day, was almost giddy as he described this new medication to our patients!

In addition to the triptans, in the chart below you will find a summary of other current medications used primarily to abort, or halt, a migraine in process.

Abortive Prescription Medications for Migraines

Medication Category	The Brand Name	Generic Form	The Good (bonuses)	The Bad (side effects)	The Ugly (precautions)
Ergotamines	Cafergot Ergomar/ Ergostat Migranal	caffeine and ergotamine sublingual ergotamine nasal ergotamine	Headache control for moderate to severe migraines	Nausea Vomiting Anxiety	Pregnant/chance of pregnancy Heart disease High blood pressure Circulation problems Vasculitis (inflammation of the blood-vessel walls)
Triptans	Imitrex Zomig Amerge Maxalt Axert Frova Relpax	sumatriptan zolmitriptan naratriptan rizatriptan almotriptan frovatriptan eletriptan	Rapid relief Available in tablet, intra-muscular injection, or nasal spray Good when vomiting is an early migraine component	Dizziness Drowsiness Nausea Weakness	Heart disease High blood pressure Taking certain antidepressants Vertebrobasilar migraine

Prescription Medications: *Anti-emetic*

I've had some migraineurs tell me they don't know what's worse, their head pain or their overwhelming nausea and repetitive vomiting they experience while in the throes (and throw-ups) of a migraine. Nausea, along with its twin sister, vomiting, can visit during a migraine headache at different times within the headache cycle. Some migraineurs get nauseous prior to their head pain, some after their head pain "gets going," and others as a result of the prescribed medication they must take in order to combat their headache. Thank the

Lord for the anti-nausea medications available on the market today! To your doctor they are known as *anti-emetic drugs*. But we can refer to them by the simpler name of *anti-nausea medication*. Taking them can send those terrible twin sisters packing.

Anti-emetic Prescription Medications for Migraines

Medication Category	The Brand Name	Generic Form	The Good (bonuses)	The Bad (side effects)	The Ugly (precautions)
Anti-emetic (anti-nausea/ vomiting)	Reglan Compazine Phenergan Promethegan Diastat	metoclopramide prochlorperazine promethazine promethazine diazepam	Available in tablet or rectally administered forms Good when severe nausea and vomiting is an early migraine component Protection from nausea side effects caused by other migraine medications	Involuntary muscle contraction Sedation	Frequent use can lead to blood abnormalities or liver disease

Prescription Medications: *Narcotic*

If you were to quietly enter the bedroom of a loved one while they were lying very still in the dark and ask, "What can I do for you?" likely they'd answer (in a low whisper), "Just make the pain stop!" That is what narcotics are for—*pain relief.* The stronger the drug is, the more effective the pain relief.

There are differing degrees of narcotic *strength* as well as *addictive potential.* The government has come up with a classification of narcotics and legal rules that govern them. As shown by the following chart, narcotics are divided into five categories, namely Schedules I through V. Schedule I drugs are found on the street—they are illegal.

Included in this category is heroin, Ecstasy, marijuana, and the like. Schedule II narcotics, which have a high potential for addiction, are strictly monitored by the government. A physician's office is not able to call in a prescription for schedule II narcotics to the pharmacy. You must have a hard-copy, paper prescription in hand when ordering them. And there are no refills without first revisiting your doctor's office and obtaining a new paper prescription. Less strictly monitored are the Schedule III narcotics. Your doctor can prescribe these for you, call the order into the pharmacy, and make refills available to you.

Schedules IV and V narcotics are not strong enough to combat migraine pain and are therefore not typically prescribed for the migraineur. One note of caution—if you have had drug or alcohol addiction problems in the past (or are presently battling one), please do yourself a huge favor and stay away from this class of drugs. The good you may get from taking them will never outweigh the risk of another addiction.

Narcotic Prescription Medications for Migraines

Medication Category	The Brand Name	Generic Form	The Good (bonuses)	The Bad (side effects)	The Ugly (precautions)
Schedule I	Illegal	–	–	Addiction	Death/overdose
Schedule II (by paper prescription only, no refills without re-evaluation by physician)	OxyContin Percocet Demerol	oxycodone oxycodone and acetaminophen meperidine	Pain relief	Constipation Dizziness Lethargy Sedation Possible addiction	Those who have had past addictive problems with drugs or alcohol Those taking other sedative medications
Schedule III (physician's office can call this into the pharmacy, refills allowed without re-evaluation)	Tylenol 3 Vicodin	acetaminophen and codeine hydrocodone and acetaminophen	Pain relief	Same as above	Same as above

Medication Category	The Brand Name	Generic Form	The Good (bonuses)	The Bad (side effects)	The Ugly (precautions)
Schedule IV	Darvon Talwin Valium Xanax	propoxyphene pentazocine diazepam alprazolam	Lower potential for addiction Not effective for migraines	Same as above	Same as above
Schedule V	Codeine-based cough medicine		Not effective for migraines	Same as above	Same as above

Cluster-Headache Management

The medical treatment of cluster-type headaches runs far behind that available to migraineurs. On the positive side, however, many cluster-headache sufferers have greatly benefited from drugs introduced to combat migraine pain, some of which are mentioned below. Let's look at what the medical field now has to offer.

Acute Therapy

Today there are two methods of treating cluster headaches. The first, *acute therapy,* refers to medications and treatments which are prescribed during an attack. This is similar to the abortive-type treatment previously discussed for migraine attacks. Below, the chart lists the most effective forms of abortive therapies presently available to cluster-headache sufferers. (I sure hope this part of my book is outdated before it even hits the market. I would rejoice alongside those who suffer with these unbearable headaches if there was an even better treatment found or medication discovered.)

The problem with the first listed therapy (the inhaled oxygen) is that by the time a cluster-headache patient makes his way to the hospital and is then *treated* in the emergency room, the headache may well be over!

Acute Therapy for Cluster Headaches

Medication Category	The Brand Name	Generic Form	The Good (bonuses)	The Bad (side effects)	The Ugly (precautions)
Oxygen	–	O_2 (100%, inhaled for 15-20 minutes)	Rapid relief for 70% of patients	–	No smoking, please
Triptans	Imitrex	Injectable sumatriptan	Rapid relief for many	Dizziness Drowsiness Nausea Weakness	Heart disease High blood pressure Taking certain antidepressants

Preventative Treatment

The second approach to treating cluster headaches is by way of *preventative treatment*. The preventative treatment approach requires daily medication dosages, which are taken in hopes of preventing or lessening the intensity of future attacks. These medicines have yielded promising results for many. There are two subgroups of preventative medications; those taken over a *short duration* and those taken *long term*.

Short-term Medications

The short-term medications, namely *corticosteroids* and *ergotamines* (see chart below), combat the swollen, inflamed blood vessels which result in the throbbing or sharp head-pain which is experienced. Because there is definite long-term side effects associated with steroid and ergotamine usage, these drugs are administered only during an existing headache-cluster period (the "active phase" of cluster headaches).

The last short-duration option listed in the chart below is a *greater occipital nerve block*. In this procedure, a mixture of a painkiller (such as lidocaine) and an anti-inflammatory medication (a steroid) is injected around the greater occipital nerve at the base of the skull. (If you recall, this nerve is "guilty" when it comes to headache production and distribution for many—see chapter 3). The results are temporary numbing of the greater occipital nerve and therefore possible headache cessation.

Short-duration Preventative Prescription Medications for Cluster Headaches

Medication Category	The Brand Name	Generic Form	The Good (bonuses)	The Bad (side effects)	The Ugly (precautions)
Corticosteroids	Prednisone Intensol Sterapred Deltasone	prednisone	Decreases inflammation	Increased appetite Weight gain Facial swelling Insomnia	Co-existing type 2 diabetes, auto-immune deficiencies, pregnancy/ breastfeeding
Ergotamines (night-time dose)	Cafergot Ergomar/ Ergostat Migranal	Caffeine and ergotamine Sublingual ergotamine Nasal ergotamine	Headache control for moderate to severe migraines	Nausea Vomiting Anxiety	Pregnant/chance of pregnancy Heart disease High blood pressure Circulation problems Vasculitis
Greater occipital nerve block		Injected lidocaine	Pain relief	–	–

Long-term Medications

Long-term preventative treatment of cluster headaches closely resembles that of migraine prevention. In fact, the same antidepressants, anti-seizure, and calcium-channel blocker medications are prescribed. Where the two headache types part company is with the *exclusion* of beta blockers as an option (which were not found to be effective with cluster headaches) and the *inclusion* of both an antipsychotic and an ergot-alkaloid medication category. (See chart below.)

Each of the five medication categories listed below all have one important thing in common: They all influence some of the chemical processes taking place in your brain (this includes the antipsychotic).

Remember the fact that you have a highly sensitive brain which magnifies incoming messages it receives and sort of blows them out of proportion, resulting in a major headache. You will hopefully find, likely by process of trial and error, that one of these medications will be effective for you. And while they will not offer you full "immunity" from cluster headaches, they may offer a shorter and softer "sentence."

Long-term Preventative Prescription Medications for Cluster Headaches

Medication Category	The Brand Name	Generic Form	The Good (bonuses)	The Bad (side effects)	The Ugly (precautions)
Antidepressants	Aventyl Elavil Pamelor Vivactil	nortriptyline amitriptyline nortriptyline protriptyline	Helpful with co-existing depression	Constipation Dry mouth Sedation Weight gain	Co-existing glaucoma, high blood pressure, and urinary retention problems
Antiseizure	Depakote Topomax	divalproex topiramate	Helpful with co-existing seizure disorders and manic-depressive illness	Fatigue Hair loss Kidney stones Nausea Tremor Weight gain	May lessen the effectiveness of oral contraceptives Pregnancy
Calcium-channel blockers	Calan Isoptin Verelan	All: verapamil	Helpful with co-existing high blood pressure	Constipation Leg swelling	Taking other heart medications
Antipsychotic	Eskalith Lithobid	lithium carbonate	Helpful with co-existing manic-depressive disorder	Drowsiness Thirst Tremor (slight) Weight gain	Precaution when taken with NSAIDs, diuretics, or high blood pressure medications Pregnancy
Ergot alkaloid	Deseril Sansert	Both: methysergide maleate	Solely used for headache control	Itching Dizziness Drowsiness Stomachache	Breastfeeding/ Pregnancy Liver, kidney, or heart disease

I hope this chapter has equipped you with the knowledge you'll need to partner with your physician as you seek medical treatment for your headaches. Always keep in mind that you are your own patient-advocate. You know yourself, your history, and your present better than anyone. Your doctor has many patients. While he or she is an expert in his or her field of medicine, you are an expert in *you*. And that, my friend, will never change.

Emotional Headaches

Chapter 12

Navigating Through the Seas of Discontent

W hat if you've tried everything and still you can't escape your headaches? You've been to all the right physicians, been treated by a great physical therapist, taken a myriad of medications, and still you find yourself suffering with head pain. I have treated many headache patients who are in the same boat as you are today. I do all the right things for them, yet their results are limited. Over the years, I have discovered a common denominator in many of these chronic head pain sufferers—*stress!*

"But Lisa, don't we all have stress?" You're quite right, we do. Stressful situations in life are inevitable. We all sail across our own personal seas of discontent from time to time. Some people's lives seem to be perpetually stormy! How then does one sail across these seas without stressing themselves into a giant headache? The survival difference between headache and nonheadache populations, as I see it, lies in their seafaring vessels and in their navigation systems. Allow me to explain.

First of all, the "starring role" that stress plays in your headaches isn't just my clinical opinion. A 2003 study published in the medical journal *Cephalgia* ("head pain"), compared a group of over 100 migraine patients with a similarly sized group of nonheadache sufferers. They found that the reported stress and anxiety levels were *significantly higher* in the migraine group. Furthermore, headache specialists and authors Young and Silberstein state, "Stress is the most common trigger for headache,"[11] and neurologists Kandel and Sudderth affirm that "stress is a major headache inducer for nearly all chronic headache types."[12]

I truly believe you can have a healing influence on your stress-induced headaches by learning how to respond differently to your stressful situations. In fact, I believe much of the stress that leads to headaches is directly related to *how you handle* what happens in your life, rather than what is actually happening.

No one is exempt from *external stress* (job loss, marital problems, rebellious teenagers, bad drivers on the road, rude people). Over these things and people you have no control. Thankfully there is something you do have control over: your *internal stress*. This is the stress of your *response* to what has occurred. It is here that your emotions and thoughts dictate your reactions. You can actually create or compound this inner form of stress by the way in which you *react* to the stormy seas you sail upon. So while you cannot control the storm surges, you can learn to control how you respond to them.

The Stress of Anger and Anxiety

Let's be real, stress is a huge subject. There are a myriad of stressful assaults you can endure and an equally large number of ways in which you can respond to them (either appropriately or inappropriately). While this is true, the two most common stormy emotions I find plaguing my headache patients are, without a doubt, *anger* and *anxiety*. These two emotions can vary from mild, appropriate responses to severe, crippling (headache-producing) manifestations.

Interestingly, your body responds to both emotions in an almost identical way. Both emotions are believed to be processed in an area of your brain called the *amygdala*. When this area of the brain is stimulated by thoughts of either anger or anxiety, chemicals are released which, in turn, create physical changes in your body. Your body's physical response to both of these emotions includes

- increased muscle tension
- increased pulse rate (heart palpitations)

- elevated blood pressure
- disturbed sleep

Hotheads and Cold Feet

The only real physical difference between an angry person and an anxious person is the temperature and electrical conductivity of their skin. During an angry episode, a person's skin temperature rises and their skin becomes more conductive. The exact opposite occurs when someone is suffering from a bout of anxiety. The anxious person's skin cools off and it becomes less conductive to electricity. Maybe this is why angry people are referred to as "hotheads" and they feel as if their anger has "ignited" them. The anxious person, conversely, reports feeling "cold and clammy" and feels as if the "spark" has gone out of them.

Keeping in mind the list of physical responses to anger and anxiety above, let's discuss why there is a significant link between these two emotions and headache production. Throughout this book I have emphasized the connection between the neck's structures and neck-related headaches as well as the role of neck dysfunction in brain-pain headaches. If you personally experience anger or anxiety, with great intensity and frequency (rather than as a fleeting, appropriate response), these emotions are creating a high "resting tone" in the muscles of your head, face, and neck areas. Have you ever gritted your teeth, clenched your jaw, or hunched your shoulders in response to either anger or anxiety? I know I have! This increased muscle tension in your head and neck aggravates the nerve endings in your muscles and can negatively affect the joints in your neck and jaw as well. As you know by now, this factor can lead to or aggravate existing headache conditions.

Elevated blood pressure and increased heart rate directly affect the vascular system in your brain. Remember the role that swollen blood vessels play in headache production? If your brain's circulation system is already highly sensitive, increasing the pressure within your vessel walls or the number of blood "pulses" sent through them can't be a good thing. Finally, disturbed sleep (or decreased time spent sleeping) is one of the headache triggers I previously highlighted in an earlier chapter. Any headache sufferer will agree that a bad night's sleep can make for an unhappy head the next day.

Dealing with Discontent

If you are someone who struggles with the powerful, headache-inducing emotions of anger and/or anxiety, be aware that there are many methods purported to aid or resolve these feelings and the physical symptoms which accompany them. Traditional intervention includes *talk therapy* and *prescription drugs* (particularly for anxiety symptoms). Talk therapy can be any form of counseling, either provided by a layperson or a professional psychotherapist/psychiatrist. Being able to verbally process your feelings and thoughts can prove quite helpful. A qualified listener will be able to offer you guidance and suggest methods of defusing and defending yourself against these forceful emotions. A psychiatrist is a licensed medical doctor who can prescribe prescription medication as well, if need be.

Alternative therapies professing to eliminate or modify the emotions of anger and anxiety are abundant and varied. (While I offer a short discussion of these, I am not endorsing any of them, as they are outside the scope of my experience with the headache population.) Studies have shown *meditation* to have an overall calming effect on a person's heart and respiration rates. It also yields a drop in muscle tension and a decrease in the circulating stress hormones in the meditator's blood stream. *Yoga* and other forms of physical exercise are often prescribed for those in need of a stress-releasing activity. Similar to meditation, they've been shown to produce positive physical results. Other varieties of alternative intervention for stress management include *acupuncture, biofeedback, aroma therapy* (for example, lavender, chamomile, and peppermint), *massage therapy,* and *herbal supplements,* such as kava kava.

The Symptom or the Root?

Something wasn't sitting right with me as I considered some of these traditional and nontraditional treatment options. What began as a vague, bothersome feeling has now materialized into a clear thought: Many of these methods, while well-meaning and even temporarily effective, are often not affecting the *root* of a person's angry or anxious feelings. Just like mowing down your dandelions produces temporary results—"Look, no weeds!"—but the next week they spring up again… all because the root remains. By only dealing with the physical signs of the dandelions, you've simply "managed" them. Their origins still remain. Likewise if you are attempting to treat anger and anxiety by dealing merely with their "after-the-fact" physical reactions and symptoms, you will never find *lasting relief.* For real relief, you must uncover and uproot the underlying cause, not just take care of their symptoms.

Well then, how does one discover the underlying, root cause of their headache-producing anger and anxiety? And is it the same root cause for everyone? It is my personal belief that there is one book which holds the answers to those two questions—the Bible. Not only does God's Word tell us *what* the root cause of anger and anxiety is, but it also offers a *cure.* In order for us to fully understand what the Bible teaches regarding the emotional "weeds" of anger and anxiety, we'll need to dig a little deeper into the soil of both stressors. Interested? Grab a shovel and we'll get started.

Acceptable Anger

Most people who are angry "by nature" or prone to angry outbursts believe their feelings and responses are justified. Just ask them. They will likely agree. (Hey, I know. I was one of them for a long time when it came to a particular area of my life.) There is always someone else to blame for their behavior. (Y'know—it's not their fault they are surrounded by a "bunch of fools"!) Seriously though, if you are willing to take an honest look at yourself, you may come to realize that anger is *your* emotional issue, as I did.

If so, it is vital for you to ask an important question regarding your anger. Which kind of anger do you have? Acceptable or destructive anger? While there are times in life when your anger may be considered acceptable, there are far more times when it is not. I find that my patients, whose headaches are triggered by an overuse of their "angry muscle," are completely unaware that this distinction even exists. They believe all of their anger is justified and therefore acceptable. Please hear me out, now. I will show you the difference between the two kinds of anger. To do so I'll use both the dictionary and the Bible.

Webster's dictionary defines anger as *a strong feeling of displeasure and usually of antagonism (opposition)*. This definition does not define anger as good or bad, simply as "what is" (as my South African friend often puts it). This is because anger isn't always a wrong response. A variation of the word anger, *indignation,* reflects just this. Indignant anger is a *righteous anger* which develops against injustice. I like to think of it as being angered by something which would anger the heart of God.

Let's look at a great example of indignation found in the Bible. It takes place in the Gospel of John, 2:13-16. This is the account of when Jesus showed up at the Temple one day and witnessed a corrupt marketplace first hand. You see, people would come from afar to worship and offer animal sacrifices to God at the temple in Jerusalem. Instead of bringing animals to be sacrificed with them from their homelands, they would bring money and purchase what they needed when they arrived at the temple. Enter the money changers and their slick sales operations. These crooks were taking advantage of out-of-town worshippers by price gouging and by using faulty scales, thus cheating them further out of their hard-earned money. And all in the name of religion...

Well, Jesus took one look at this "farmers' market" and got angry. So very angry that he made a whip out of cords and slung it at the market's tables overturning them, spilling their contents to the ground and scattering animals everywhere. Now Jesus, the Bible tells us, was a man who was without sin. So we can deduce that his angry outburst was devoid of wrongdoing and therefore acceptable in his Father's sight.

While it is true that there are occasions in which anger is "right" before God, his Word specifically cautions us against *un*righteous anger by warning us in Ephesians 4:26, "In your anger do not sin." This verse is cautioning us against the second and more common type of anger: destructive.

Destructive Anger

How then does anger become unrighteous (sinful) and destructive to ourselves and to those around us? I believe it has to do with *who* is at the center of the anger. In the above section we looked at a biblical example in which God and his laws were treated with disdain and carelessness. Therefore, the anger displayed was God-centered and based upon violation of his laws. Where I believe you and I err, and enter into destructive anger, is when *we* are at the center of our anger. A negative outcome (and possible headache) is sure to result when we get angry and act out (or seethe) because

- our rights (as we see them) have been violated
- our (precious) time has been wasted
- our (most important) self has been insulted.

By behaving in this manner, we become the judge over our circumstances, deciding which annoyance or insult requires an angry response from us. Because we act as our own judge and jury, this means there are no absolute standards of right and wrong responses, only subjective ones. Often our responses change on a day-to-day basis. Our self-determined "righteous" anger depends solely upon how we judged what just happened. Rather than being God-centered, this destructive response is self-centered and self-justified.

The Bible has much to say about this self-driven response. Ecclesiastes 7:9 warns us, "Do not be quickly provoked in your spirit, for anger resides in the lap of fools." Proverbs 29:11 tells us: "A fool gives full vent to his anger, but a wise man keeps himself under control" and Colossians 3:8 says to "rid yourself of anger and rage." God, the Creator, knows what makes you tick, and he knows what makes you sick. For your benefit he has revealed His will for your life (and your responses) through his holy Scriptures. Our physical health often depends upon how well we take his Word to heart.

Can anyone keep him or herself out of destructive anger completely? No, not on this side of heaven. But we can make progress and we can find help. Before we get to that critical help though, let's complete our study of stressful emotions by taking a revealing look at anxiety. Afterwards, we will go directly to the Bible in search of help and healing.

Anxiety That Stresses You Out

The word *anxiety* is often used interchangeably with the words *fear* and *worry*. Webster's dictionary classifies it as

An abnormal and overwhelming sense of apprehension and fear often marked by:

1. physiological signs (sweating, tension, and increased pulse rate),

2. doubt concerning the reality and nature of the threat, and

3. self-doubt about one's capacity to cope with it.

Anxiety is synonymous with "uncontrolled worrying." Interestingly, the original word for *worry* in the Old High German is the word *würgen*, which means "to choke or strangle." If you have ever been overcome by anxious thoughts, you may have felt just that...a choking sensation or a tightening around your throat.

Anxiety That Works

Anxiety, by definition, seems to get a purely bad rap. It would appear that nothing good can come of it. On the contrary, there is a mild form that is known by performers, athletes, and the like as *performance anxiety.* This light form of anxiety actually improves a person's performance by slightly increasing their blood flow, increasing their level of alertness (focus), and increasing the response-time of their muscles.

You are certainly not alone if you find yourself struggling with feelings of anxiety. Anxiety disorders are the most common mental illness in the United States. Forty million (18.1 percent) of the adult population (those aged 18 and older) are affected! Anxiety occurs in different intensities and with various manifestations. General anxiety disorders (GAD) are the most common form of anxiety problems. When anxiety gets further "out of control," it manifests itself as panic attacks, obsessive-compulsive disorders, post-traumatic stress disorders, and other assorted phobias.

If you're having trouble finding relief from your headaches (after all we've already covered), and you know anxiety is a storm which continues to batter against your vessel, there is a lifeboat within reach. Follow me as I share my personal journey from stressful sailing to peaceful passage.

Who's to Blame?

Many people claim that they "just can't help it" when it comes to feeling angered or anxious. Believe me when I say "I've been there." For many years I struggled with anger which, given the right circumstances, would flare up into rage (typically at my father). I was hurt and felt I was justified in hurting him back with my anger.

In addition to my problem with anger, I've also suffered through anxious periods as well—those which have tightened up my throat, the muscles in my chest, head, neck, and shoulders, and have led me straight into a throbbing headache. In fact, a few years ago I was at the mercy of multiple storms which converged on my boat simultaneously. Following a serious medical diagnosis of my daughter, an unexpected surgery for my son, a difficult situation concerning my mom's mental illness, as well as a serious look at relocating our family to another state, my throat closed up so tightly, I nearly had to visit the emergency department at the local hospital.

This anxious state lasted for many months. Through it all, God gently and graciously taught me life-changing lessons regarding my anger and times of prolonged anxiety, and I am truly "anxious" to share them with you.

I have a growing faith in Jesus Christ. Through years of reading and studying my Bible, daily prayer, the counsel of godly friends, and after countless sermon teachings, God has revealed an important truth about my anger (which may be true of you too). Whenever I hold unrighteous anger in my heart, it exposes my belief that...

- *I* am of primary importance. (More important than who or what I am mad at.)
- *I* should receive first class treatment and consideration.
- *My* time and *my* schedule are more important than those around me.
- *My* feelings reign supreme.

I came to understand that by behaving in this way, I was relying on my angry outbursts to "make things right," rather than relying on God to work out all things for my good (Romans 8:28). Furthermore, by acting as the protector of my rights, I was not allowing God to be my Protector. Romans 12:19 reads, "Do not take revenge, my friends, but leave room for God's wrath (his righteous anger), for it is written: 'It is mine to avenge; I will repay,' says the Lord." You see, if we have been unjustly treated, God is on our side and he wants to be the one to make things right for us. Over time, I've learned to leave the "protecting job" to him.

The second thing I've come to understand (and continue to learn to apply) is that when I find myself in a prolonged period of anxiety, I am guilty of believing that God can't or won't handle my future in a way that is in my best interest. If this belief were not true, why else would I be in angst over something that God has already promised to sustain me through (Psalm 55:22)? The Word of God clearly demonstrates that the root cause for *every* person's destructive anger and anxiety are the same as mine if you boil them down to their essence: limited trust in God.

This was quite a blow of realization for me. As humans we hate to take the blame for anything, especially when someone or something else can be easily blamed instead. The truth is, you and I must take responsibility for how we respond to the stressful storms which roll across our seas and threaten our peace—no matter what our circumstances are or were. The exciting thing is, once we understand the underlying sources of our emotional responses, we can act to do something about it.

Consider this—by giving in to the destructive responses of anger and anxiety as I sailed across my Seas of Discontent, I had, in effect, launched out in my own "dinghy," trying to ride through the storms of my life by using my own defensive strategies. In doing so, I abandoned God's seaworthy vessel (complete with navigation system—the Bible). So in answer to my own question: "Who's to blame?" I'd have to admit, *I am.* The Bible clearly instructs me to "be anxious for nothing" (Philippians 4:6-9) and to "put away all anger" (paraphrased from Ephesians 4:31). It opposes God's character to make a commandment against something I am powerless to change. His Word confirms that I have a choice in the matters of anger and anxiety. Faced with that knowledge, I had a decision to make.

Changing Your Outlook to an "Uplook"

Those who know me best would say that today my life is characterized by *peace* rather than by the destructive emotions of anger and anxiety. How was I able to make this change? Author Beth Moore explains it best in her book *Living Beyond Yourself,* when she writes, "We cannot possibly experience the peace *of* God until we have peace *with* God."

My peace with God initially began with an action on my part. I had to confess to God that my anger and my anxious thoughts were sinful and self-centered, according to the Bible. Once I confessed my guilt and asked God for forgiveness, I had to ask for something else: his power to respond to the stresses of my life differently—in ways that pleased his heart, rather than grieved his heart.

The first step I took brought me peace with God. The second step continues to bring me peace with others and with myself. Certainly this second part is a process. But just as practice improves performance, my responses have been improving with each new challenge. Sometimes, however, I flat out fail. But when I do, I begin back at step one and I make peace with God (through confession). I follow up with making peace with anyone I have offended (admitting my wrongful response and asking them for forgiveness). Then I cast my eyes upward again and sail on.

By changing my "outlook" to an "uplook" in the areas of anger and anxiety, I have found a new way to navigate through my Seas of Discontent. It is on the ship of my Savior, Jesus Christ. I have put my full trust in him. He is my protector (from wrongs done against me), and he is my future holder (and therefore, anxiety-reducer). Jeremiah 29:11 reveals God's heart for mankind: "I know the plans I have for you, declares the LORD, plans to prosper you and not to harm you, plans to give you hope and a future."

Peaceful Passages

Jesus tells us in the gospel of John 14:27, "*My* peace I give you... Do not let your hearts be troubled and do not be afraid." Look at the emphasized word in that verse. Jesus is offering us *his* peace. It belongs to him, yet he is giving it to us. What Jesus is offering to us is the very peace of God...a relief from anxiety and anger. That was a gift I simply could no longer refuse to accept. I love the words of King Solomon in Proverbs 14:30: "A heart at peace brings life to the body." We definitely know the opposite can be true, don't we? A heart full of anger or anxiety diminishes our health and gives us—among other things—headaches.

God does not promise us that he will calm the "storms" on our seas, but he will provide a protective covering. It's often said, "God is not a bridge over troubled waters, he is a tunnel through them." This reflects Jesus' words to us in John 16:33 when he encouraged us by saying, "In this world you will have trouble. But take heart! I have overcome the world." The truth is we can have God's peace in the midst of distressing circumstances. By trusting in God's promises, we can have the complete assurance that we are under his watchful eye and in the palm of his caring hand all the while.

If you are interested in "jumping ship" (onto his worthy vessel), pray with intent the prayer found on page 193. Yes, it is as easy as that. He will answer your honest prayer and you will have peace *with* God. Then the peace *of* God can be yours today.

Prayer

Dear Lord Jesus,

I acknowledge I am a sinner. I've completely missed the mark,
and I need a Savior—someone to completely transform my life.

I thank you for paying the price for my sins.

By dying on the cross,
you took care of all my failures, all my unwholesome acts,
and all the ways I tried to be my own god.

I accept your gift of forgiveness and eternal life—
new life that begins now and lasts forever with you in heaven.

In the same power that God used to resurrect you from the grave,
I declare that my old self has been made new.

I give you full control of my life.

Make me into the person you designed me to be.

And now I want my new life to reflect you and show forth how good
you are.

In Jesus' name,

Amen.

Finally, be blessed, my friend.
It was a privilege to walk beside you on this journey to healing.
I trust better days are on your horizon.

AMERICAN ACADEMY OF NEUROLOGY FOUNDATION
1080 Montreal Avenue
Saint Paul, MN 55116
www.aan.com

The AAN is the world's leading organization of neurology professionals and a strong advocate of public education, as reflected by its affiliated site, www.thebrainmatters.org. The AAN site itself is primarily for its physician members.

The Web site *www.thebrainmatters.org* is an excellent educational resource that provides information on a variety of topics related to migraine and other neurologic disorders. It is the patient education site of the American Academy of Neurology Foundation.

AMERICAN COUNCIL FOR HEADACHE EDUCATION (ACHE)
19 Mantua Road
Mt. Royal, NJ 08061
Tel: 856-423-0258; 800-255-ACHE (255-2243)
Fax: 856-423-0082
achehq@talley.com
www.achnet.org

ACHE is a nonprofit patient-health professional partnership dedicated to advancing the treatment and management of headache and to raising the public awareness of headache as a valid, biologically based illness. Its goals are to empower headache sufferers through education, and to support them by educating their families, employers, and the public in general.

ACHE was created in 1990 through an initiative of the American Headache Society (see below). Its Web site has extensive resource information, a listing of support groups, and much more.

AMERICAN HEADACHE SOCIETY
19 Mantua Road
Mt. Royal, NJ 08061
Tel: 856-423-0043
Fax: 856-423-0082
ahshq@talley.com
www.ahsnet.org

The American Headache Society (AHS) is an organization of more than 2400 physicians, health professionals, and research scientists. Its Web site contains information primarily of interest to clinical professionals; this organization works closely with ACHE to produce educational programs and materials, coordinate its support groups, and undertake public awareness initiatives.

NATIONAL HEADACHE FOUNDATION
820 N. Orleans, Suite 217
Chicago, IL 60610-3132
Tel: 773-388-6399; 888-NHF-5552 (643-5552)
Fax: 773-525-7357
info@headaches.org
www.headaches.org

The foundation's goals are to serve as an information resource to headache sufferers, their families, and the health-care providers who treat them; to raise public awareness that headaches are a legitimate biological disease and sufferers should receive understanding and continuity of care; and to promote research into potential headache causes and treatments.

The foundation Web site offers information on a variety of topics related to headache, information on support groups, information about clinical trials, publications, and much more.*

Notes

1. Actual statistics are unreliable. Some studies will state 1 patient in 1 million will have adverse affects to upper neck joint thrusts, but *reporting* of such incidents is questionable, as Dr. Edzard Ernst found in his survey. In total, 35 cases had been seen by the 24 neurologists who responded, *but none of the cases had been reported*. He concluded that underreporting in the medical literature was close to 100 percent, rendering estimates "nonsensical." See Edzard Ernst, "Spinal Manipulation: Its safety is uncertain" *Etc.*, January 8, 2002, p. 166. In the article, Ernst makes reference to C. Stevenson, W. Honan, B. Cooke, and E. Ernst, "Neurological complications of cervical spine manipulation," *Journal of the Royal Society of Medicine,* 2001:94, pp. 107-110.

2. Ernst, "Spinal Manipulation," p. 166, emphasis added.

3. Richard P. DiFabio, "Manipulation of the Cervical Spine: risks and benefits," *Physical Therapy* magazine, 1999:79 (1), pp. 50-65. This article was a review of the scientific literature on the risks and benefits of manipulation of the cervical spine (MCS). The 177 cases DiFabio reviewed were reported in 116 articles published between 1925 and 1997. Special care was taken, whenever possible, to correctly identify all the professions responsible for any injuries and/or deaths.

4. DiFabio.

5. DiFabio.

6. DiFabio.

7. DiFabio.

8. Adapted from David Buchholz, MD, *Heal Your Headache* (New York: Workman Publishing, 2002), pp. 74-75; and Teri Robert, *Living Well with Migraine Disease and Headaches* (New York: HarperCollins Publishers, 2005), p. 110-111.

9. Adapted from Buchholz, pp. 38,40-41,112-113,189.

10. William B. Young, MD, and Stephen D. Silberstein, MD, *Migraine and Other Headaches* (New York: AAN Press, 2004), pp. 81-101, 133, 135.

11. Young and Silberstein, p. 53.

12. Joseph Kandel, MD, and David Sudderth, MD, *The Headache Cure* (New York: McGraw-Hill, 2006), pp. 186-187.

About the Author

Lisa Morrone graduated magna cum laude from the physical therapy program at the State University of New York at Stony Brook in 1989, receiving a Bachelor of Science degree in Physical Therapy. In addition to her college education, Lisa has taken over 30 continuing education courses in the area of orthopedic physical therapy. As a physical therapist, Lisa has been treating patients in the field of orthopedic rehabilitation for nearly two decades. In 1990 she accepted the position of adjunct professor at Touro College, Bay Shore, New York, which she still holds today.

At Touro College Lisa instructs in both the Entry Level and the Post-Professional Doctorate Programs in Physical Therapy. Presently Lisa co-teaches Musculoskeletal II (Spinal Orthopedics), Spinal Stabilization Training (core strengthening of the trunk, hips, and shoulder-blade muscles), and an advanced elective on Spinal Muscle Energy Techniques (evaluation and treatment specific to the spinal joints). Her past teaching credits also include: Massage, Extremity Joint Mobilization (evaluation and treatment of the joints in the arms and legs), and Kinesiology (the study of bones, muscles, and joints and their roles in the human body).

Lisa's first book, *Overcoming Back and Neck Pain,* was published in February 2007. Lisa is a graduate of both the speaker and the writer tracks of the She Speaks Conference (Proverbs 31 Ministries), where she was assessed at the highest level of proficiency. As a speaker, Lisa has taught in both secular (community and medical) and church-based settings. She makes her home on Long Island, New York along with her husband, daughter, and son.

Restoring Your Temple™

Within Christian circles, one's physical body is often referred to as the temple of the Holy Spirit. The reason for this is found in 1 Corinthians 6:19, where the Bible says, "Do you not know that your body is a temple of the Holy Spirit, who is in you, whom you have received from God?" Temples are places where worship takes place. But what exactly is worship? To quote author Rick Warren,

> Worship is far more than praising, singing, and praying to God. Worship is a lifestyle of *enjoying* God, *loving* him and *giving* ourselves to be used for his purposes. When you use your life for God's glory, everything you do can become an act of worship.

Romans 12:1 further tells us to "offer your *bodies* as living sacrifices, holy and pleasing to God—this is your spiritual act of worship." God has plans for your body…physical plans. Your hands and feet are meant to be used as his hands and feet on this earth. So whether he calls you to raise children, teach Sunday school, or work with teenagers or the homeless, you need a physical body that is ready for action. Scripture says, "The harvest is plentiful, but the workers are few." Oftentimes this is because the workers are at a doctor's appointment, going to physical therapy, or are simply so tired they can't get off the couch!

It is the intent of **Restoring Your Temple** to ready the Body of Christ to perform the work of Christ. The longer you live in good physical health, the more you will be able to enjoy the abundant life God has promised to his children.

Visit Lisa Morrone's Web site, **www.RestoringYourTemple.com,** for

- downloadable headache charts
- dietary trigger list
- a home exercise program for those suffering with jaw pain (TMD)
- further help with issues of physical health and well-being
- a source of "Lisa-tested," quality health-related products
- quick tips for back, neck, head, or jaw pain
- guidance on how to find a good physical therapist
- Lisa's personal testimony

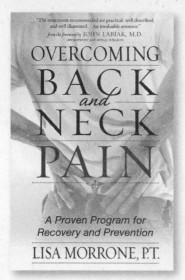

OVERCOMING BACK AND NECK PAIN

A Proven Program for Recovery and Prevention

"The treatments Lisa recommends are practical, well described, and well illustrated...An invaluable resource."

FROM THE FOREWORD BY JOHN LABIAK, MD, ORTHOPAEDIST AND SPINAL SURGEON

Do you want to get out of pain and enjoy your life again?

From 20 years of teaching and practicing physical therapy, Lisa Morrone gives you a way to say no to the treadmill of prescriptions, endless treatments, and a limited lifestyle. This straightforward, clinically proven approach offers the most effective exercises, guidelines, and lifestyle adjustments for back and neck problems, showing you how to...

- benefit from good posture and "core stability"
- strengthen and stretch key muscles
- shift to healthy movement patterns
- recover from pain caused by compressed or degenerated discs
- address "inside issues" that affect your body's healing capacity— nutrition, rest, and emotional/spiritual struggles

With Lisa's help, you can gain freedom from pain—and regain your freedom to enjoy work, friends, family, and a fulfilling life.

"This book takes a very practical approach to the key things patients really need to know."

KENT KEYSER, MS, PT, OCS, COMT, ATC, FFCFMT, FAAOMPT
PRACTICING AND TEACHING PHYSICAL THERAPIST

To read a chapter from this or any other Harvest House book, go to www.harvesthousepublishers.com.

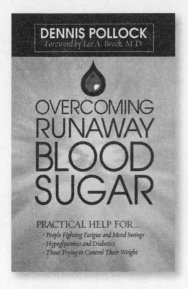

OVERCOMING RUNAWAY BLOOD SUGAR
Dennis Pollock

Want to gain energy, lose weight, and enjoy better health? With this positive, can-do approach, you can gain maximum health while losing excess pounds. You'll discover...

- why runaway blood sugar is a key factor in food cravings and weight issues
- how blood-sugar problems lead to damage to your body
- ways to evaluate pre-diabetes health risks, such as hypoglycemia
- reasons and motivation to change your lifestyle
- diet and exercise that really work

Whether you are diabetic, have a family history of diabetes, or are simply tired of being sick and tired, *Overcoming Runaway Blood Sugar* may very well change the way you view eating and exercise forever.

To read a chapter from this or any other Harvest House book,
go to www.harvesthousepublishers.com.

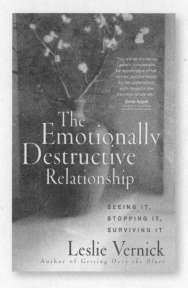

THE EMOTIONALLY DESTRUCTIVE RELATIONSHIP
Seeing It, Stopping It, Surviving It

Leslie Vernick

Stop. Dare to ask the question: What's going wrong in this relationship?

Maybe it doesn't seem to be "abuse." No bruises, no sexual violation. Even smiles on the surface. Nonetheless, before your eyes, a person is being destroyed emotionally. Perhaps that person is someone you want to help. Perhaps it's you.

Step by step, author and counselor Leslie Vernick guides you on how to…

- recognize behaviors that are meant to control, punish, and hurt
- confront and speak truth when the timing is right
- determine when to keep trying and when to shift your approach
- get safe and stay safe
- continue your relationship with God

Do you want to change? Within the pages of this book, you will find spiritually sound, straightforward help to take the first step today.

To read a chapter from this or any other Harvest House book,
go to www.harvesthousepublishers.com.

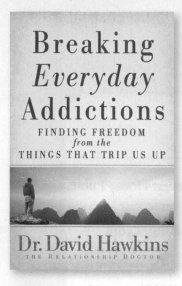

BREAKING EVERYDAY ADDICTIONS

Finding Freedom from the Things That Trip Us Up

Dr. David Hawkins

*You know you have a problem...*but what can you do about it? You've tried going for a few days without drinking coffee, checking your e-mails, or watching TV, but your good intentions seem to get you only so far.

This eye-opening book reveals that such repeated behaviors can easily become true addictions that control you and limit your ability to make good choices. But help is available—even if you or a loved one struggle with a more destructive behavior. *Breaking Everyday Addictions* shows you how God can lead you to freedom and points you to up-to-date answers for questions like these:

- Is addiction a disease? If it is, are addicts responsible for their behavior?
- Why do anorexics and morbidly obese people continue their self-destructive behavior?
- What is the appeal of gambling against nearly unbeatable odds?

Breaking free from addictions isn't easy. But with the information and practical steps Dr. Hawkins provides, you can create a program of recovery that will help you and the people you love regain control and build happier, healthier lives.

To read a chapter from this or any other Harvest House book, go to www.harvesthousepublishers.com.

hers
:

DATE DUE
